Praise for

SATTVA

'Eminé and Paul both strive to live and breathe what they preach with absolute grace. Sattva, and the tools to live a conscious, harmonious life, are never more important than in the busy, overwhelming world we now find ourselves in.'

JASMINE HEMSLEY, CO-FOUNDER OF HEMSLEY & HEMSLEY, AUTHOR OF *EAST BY WEST* AND CO-AUTHOR OF *THE ART OF EATING WELL*

'If you are looking for a way to free yourself from anxiety, stress and speed then I recommend you read Eminé and Paul Rushton's book, Sattva. It is a guide to good living. The authors weave together the ancient philosophy of India with practical advice for our time. Practising the principals described in Sattva will lead you to live a simple, fulfilling and meaningful life. The book is full of inspiring thoughts and helpful tips for daily action. It is a wonderful contribution to the literature about personal and planetary wellbeing.'

SATISH KUMAR, PEACE AND ENVIRONMENT ACTIVIST, AUTHOR AND FORMER EDITOR OF *RESURGENCE & ECOLOGIST* MAGAZINE

'Whether you want to dive right into the Ayurvedic lifestyle or you simply want to add a few elements of calm to your life, Eminé and Paul are the best guides. By immersing themselves in the Vedic life, they have distilled all the wisdom you need to make your journey to peace and sattva calm and easy.'

BRIGID MOSS, CONTRIBUTING HEALTH DIRECTOR, *RED* MAGAZINE

'I've been following Eminé's journey – online and in real life – since we met six years ago. She writes straight from the heart, which is completely captivating, honest, vulnerable and relatable. Since I've known her, at first professionally and then as a great friend, I've always saved her emails, advice and Instagram posts. Now, finally, she has her wisdom, her learnings and her journey in one wonderful book which I will keep close by and enjoy whenever I want. Eminé is the best reminder to carve out some peace and time for tea everyday for yourself.'

MELISSA HEMSLEY, CO-FOUNDER OF HEMSLEY & HEMSLEY AND AUTHOR OF EAT HAPPY

'Eminé and Paul have managed to write a book about an ancient medical system in a language that is not only easy to understand but also inspiring. The gentle tone of the book inspires you to want to live a more balanced and conscious life.'

NADIA NARAIN, YOGA TEACHER AND CO-AUTHOR OF SELF CARE FOR THE REAL WORLD

'Eminé and Paul are inspired and inspiring. They have translated the ancient science of Ayurveda into a language of sweet simplicity. Sattva is a blissful benediction, a blueprint for soulful living in a frenzied world. I can't recommend it highly enough.'

JANE ALEXANDER, HEALTH AND WELLBEING JOURNALIST, AND AUTHOR OF SPIRIT OF THE HOME

'Sattva beautifully encapsulates the essence of the ancient Vedic teachings to truly live consciously in our busy modern world. This book is accessible and practical, and an essential read for anyone on a journey of self discovery and a quest to find true harmony.'

GEETA VARA, AYURVEDIC PRACTITIONER AND AUTHOR OF AYURVEDA

'The moment I opened Sattva it was like breathing in a deep breath of tranquillity and peace – pure medicine for the soul. This book is an important and fundamental requirement for our physical health and inner wellbeing today, to counteract the impact our fast-paced, modern-day lives are having on our mind, body, heart and soul. Filled with so much wisdom and practical guidance on how we can all live more consciously, connected, grounded and in tune, Sattva needs to be on every book shelf and part of everyone's lives today.'

NICKY CLINCH, TRANSFORMATIONAL COACH, SPIRITUAL MENTOR AND FOUNDER OF THE WARRIOR WOMAN MOVEMENT

'Leading from their hearts, on a foundation of love and gratitude, and with light shining from their souls, Eminé and Paul have given us a truly conscious guide to thrive. This modern wisdom offers needed respite in this hectic world. Every thought expressed poignantly and delivered with such passion, intention and integrity.'

ANNEE DE MAMIEL, FOUNDER OF DE MAMIEL

'Walking in the path of the ever-emerging mystery of life brings up many feelings and questions. What could be better than learning more about sattva – the path to literally knowing your own truth – on this remarkable journey? In this book of insights into the meaning and experience of sattva, you will find many pertinent gems to inspire you on your way.'

SEBASTIAN POLE, CO-FOUNDER OF PUKKA HERBS AND AUTHOR OF *A PUKKA LIFE*

'This is truly wonderful wisdom to put into the world at this time. Eastern medicine is dear to my heart, and we can learn so much from this deeply observational medicine, and this utterly beautiful book.'

EMMA CANNON, LEADING WOMEN'S WELLBEING EXPERT AND AUTHOR OF *FERTILE*

'Eminé and Paul haven't just written a beautiful book, they have lived and learned every single word of its pages. It is a privilege to have this in my hands, to learn from what they have so eloquently shared with us in Sattva.'

ANNIE CLARKE, FOUNDER AND AUTHOR OF *MIND BODY BOWL*

SATTVA

SATTVA

The Ayurvedic Way
to Live Well

EMINÉ & PAUL RUSHTON

HAY HOUSE

Carlsbad, California • New York City
London • Sydney • New Delhi

Published in the United Kingdom by:
Hay House UK Ltd, The Sixth Floor, Watson House
54 Baker Street, London W1U 7BU
Tel: +44 (0)20 3927 7290; Fax: +44 (0)20 3927 7291; www.hayhouse.co.uk

Published in Australia by:
Hay House Australia Ltd, 18/36 Ralph St, Alexandria NSW 2015
Tel: (61) 2 9669 4299; Fax: (61) 2 9669 4144; www.hayhouse.com.au

Published in India by:
Hay House Publishers India, Muskaan Complex, Plot No.3, B-2,
Vasant Kunj, New Delhi 110 070
Tel: (91) 11 4176 1620; Fax: (91) 11 4176 1630; www.hayhouse.co.in

A catalogue record for this book is available from the British Library.

Hardcover ISBN: 978-1-78817-224-0
E-book ISBN: 978-1-78817-307-0
Audiobook ISBN: 978-1-78817-372-8

Interior images: Alisha Kruger of Love Indigo Creative

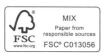

MIX
Paper from
responsible sources
FSC
www.fsc.org   FSC® C013056

Printed and bound in Great Britain by
TJ International Ltd, Padstow, Cornwall

To our most beloved teachers,
Mia Anaïs and Celie June,
We love you the sun,
We love you the moon.

'Sattva is the quality of light, love and life, the higher or spiritual force that allows us to evolve in consciousness.'

DR DAVID FRAWLEY

YOGA & AYURVEDA: SELF-HEALING AND SELF-REALIZATION

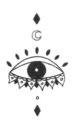

CONTENTS

SATTVA

INTRODUCTION

Sattva: In Sanskrit: 'consciousness'.

Definition: the quality of goodness – love, light and
a life lived well; rich in peace, selflessness, serenity,
enlightenment, gentleness and harmony.

S O MUCH OF MODERN LIFE IS LIVED LOST AMONG THE TREES – no wood
in sight. The bigger picture blurred by the bleeping phone and
the flashing screen, the breathless commute, the howl of the baby. Life
involves a lot of getting up and getting on. We exist on the back foot: just
about head-above-water and in a relentless state of minor panic, 'fight or
flight'… reactive rather than responsive.

We've been living this way for far too long. Perhaps it began with the
first modem or smartphone; with the immediacy of social media, the
red-eye flight or the first direct message; the thrumming fluorescent
light or the clamour of the 24-hour supermarket. But at some point, we

forgot that we weren't made to be always 'on'; that our 'out of office' would become a mere smokescreen, since we would continue to respond to those 'urgent' emails even while marooned on a desert island (with exceptional Wi-Fi).

We've seen the rise in anxiety, and stress-related disorders; the rise in insomnia; the rise in diabetes and heart disease. We're flooded with awareness of the fact that our lifestyles are making us ill – the pace and pressure and permanence of it all: utterly unrelenting, wholly unsustainable.

History has taught us that the greatest change and the most profound social progress are often made in direct response to chaos, confusion, pain, tragedy. Nadirs of darkness and shame are overtaken by periods of dazzling political and social renaissance: the power of the pendulum, as we try to right the wrongs and learn from our mistakes. It takes a whole lot of us to wake up, rise up and declare 'no more!' before anything really changes. And that is precisely what's beginning to happen: right here, right now.

ANOTHER WAY OF LIVING

Because, all along, there has been a way of living that supports our own intuition; that connects each of us with the big picture, in every single way, every single day. A way of living that sees the whole and the whole of us: the moon, sky, sun, sea, stars, breath, body, spirit and mind. A way of encompassing all the most minute, dearest elements of our selves – every atom of being and whisper of breath – into one harmonious, indistinguishably complete picture. It's a truly holistic state where peace, harmony, connectedness and ease prevail.

We're increasingly beginning to invite those things that we know, deep down inside, will bring us contentment, peace, ease: *wellbeing*. We're talking about self-care with unprecedented vigour and beginning to see it for the radical act it really is. Why? Because nothing has a greater impact on the wellbeing of others than our own wellbeing.

At peace within our selves, we radiate that peace outwards. We go into our daily interactions with love and compassion; we're present and giving; we share kindness as freely as the air we breathe. When all is well within us, we feel as though all is well around us, or that we're less porous, somehow, to the ill winds when it's not.

We're waking up. All around, there's a slow movement emerging – a natural return to the simple beauty of 'being' – and a conscious move away from relentless 'overdoing'. We're increasingly meditating and practising mindfulness; shelving the smartphone for a while to plait wreaths, carve spoons or take up calligraphy; we're swapping our brutal boot camp weekends for self-love circles, and our punishing, calorie-counting runs for hyggelig cinnamon buns.

We're becoming warier of how much we buy and throw away, and increasingly choosing to make, grow, bake and mend. We're seeing a return to these gentle trends – mindful medicine for the mindless malady – because our very best instincts are leading us there. We're also feeling a shift away from the *see* of heavily processed convenience food and the *saw* of raw, cold and squeaky clean – to deeply nourishing, whole and enticing bowls of simmered seasonal goodness to be savoured and absorbed; from Insta-perfect pin-ups of washboard abdominals, to honest, soft and exquisite celebrations of divine femininity.

We've become sceptical of the virtues of working ourselves into the ground, and many of us now seek instead the alignment of our work with our values – our *dharma*: following the heart over the mind. We've grown increasingly weary and wary of the mushrooming digital world, and are finding more answers within. A revolution is beginning (and it will not be televised).

A Return to Our Intuition

Deeply at the heart of it all, many of us are beginning to think about ourselves as *spiritual* beings. That we ever stopped doing so is the saddest part of all. For tens of thousands of years of human history, we've lived lives rich in ceremony, ritual and colour. We've given thanks, attributed meaning, sat in silence under skies full of stars and breath-rescinding natural vistas, appreciated and savoured.

Introduction

For millennia we've been instinctive and open – wholly tuned in. We're a race of beings who once recognized and responded to our needs so naturally, that the idea of *not* doing so would've been lost in translation: anathema. Our entire relationship with our selves was self-care. We thrived as a species because our intuition guided us well – we sought truth, told stories, slept and replenished. We hunted and gathered. We made love and followed the stars. We painted our caves and made jewellery. Every day, we greeted the rising sun with the exuberance of all the other creatures; we ebbed with the dusk and flowed with the dawn.

We've long left the cave behind, but in the thoroughly modern, technicolour, surround sound, simulcast present day, we need 'the simple life' more than ever. And, although 5,000 years ago the lifestyle choices we made were very different, there are fundamental principles of living well that carry over to all of us – regardless of geography or history – via the common threads we all share: our humanity and our consciousness.

We're at the very onset of a time of significant, necessary, healing change, and this 'shift' that so many of us are presently feeling, is rooted in something deeply profound, ancient and true. This growing 'awareness' comes as a direct result of the challenge and chaos that has preceded it – from rising symptoms like Trump and Brexit, ecological breakdown and mass extinction, to cultural fear, unconscious consumerism and endless social media consumption. Out of the chaos, comes a return to conscious living. Thank goodness, then, for sattva.

WHY SATTVA?

Sattva is a Sanskrit word that means both mind and consciousness; *sat*, too, means truth. Sattva is the purest essence of goodness – an awakened life, peaceful mind, vital body, pure spirit. It's a core concept within Vedic science – of which Ayurveda and Yoga are both sister sciences. Ayurveda is a traditional system of health care that originated in India in ancient times and is still widely practised across India, in parts of Asia and increasingly so in the West; and Yoga is one of the six systems (*darshans*) of Indian philosophy and the foundation of a life well-lived.

Sattva is a 'feeling' and an energy: a primal quality and natural force that enters every part of our lives – from restful, worry-free sattvic sleep, to gentle, easily digested and vital sattvic suppers. It's the knowledge of life as it truly is: clear as day, light and love-filled.

Sattva is a word that's found, over and over, within Vedic and yogic texts, and it's one that we found ourselves using more and more as we tried to explain the quality or 'feeling' of life that we felt so intuitively drawn to. But it also, so succinctly and poetically, encompasses all the qualities of 'living well' that felt so right to us, without our questioning why.

As a young family, we knew we'd been making ever-more conscious choices: from the food we grow and the tiny swatches of land we sustain, to the sustainable clothes, barefoot shoes and natural personal care products we select for ourselves and our children. And we knew that our choices had to 'feel good' – aligned with our wish to live in a gentle, loving, ethical way – in order to invite good energy back into our lives.

We started to forgo television at night in favour of sitting out on the doorstep of our little terraced cottage, sheltered by towering evergreens, sipping tea beneath a canopy of stars and moonlight. We were rising before the sun to a gentle meditation, a cup of chai and a slow unravelling of thoughts. It was a stark contrast to the chaotic commute and sleep-deprived baby years we'd known several years earlier.

People became curious – they felt a shift, we think, and wanted to know what had changed. It wasn't something we could immediately put our fingers on. One small, conscious choice begot another, all with one thing uniting them – a wish to live a simpler, lighter, freer, gentler life. Again – a *feeling* much more than a thought; being over doing.

Out of this feeling arose conscious movement – towards a life that felt good each and every day – and while there were, and will yet be, many stumbles along the path, the righting of the wrong-footedness became ever easier, ever subtler, ever more natural.

So... having lived in accordance with Ayurveda for the best part of a decade, one sunny afternoon at our local community café and Yoga studio in Kent, we sat quietly, side by side, *feeling* into a word that might amply express all the conscious choices, emotions, experiences and knowledge that had paved our path to that point. We both reached for a piece of paper and wrote down the same word at the same time: SATTVA. *That* is when this book truly began.

VEDIC SCIENCE – HOME OF YOGA AND AYURVEDA

What we trust, so very deeply, is that regardless of time, space, geography and culture, *truth is truth*. Sattva cannot be created or destroyed – it's a primal quality and energy, after all – but while it exists all around us, we can only benefit from it when we actively seek it out and invite it into our lives.

To eradicate pain and suffering we must disempower the ego and silence the mind; but in order to do this, we have to work on transcending them both – on rising above the petty thoughts and self-limiting beliefs to a place where we tap into our highest and purest levels of consciousness.

Five thousand years ago, a wise, devoted *rishi* (seer or sage) who sat in deepest meditation, chanting Vedic mantra, might have experienced sattva to the point of *samhadi*: purest, highest consciousness. He did so not to become an enlightened, awakened, empowered individual (there's that ego again), but in order to liberate himself completely from all thoughts of a disconnected 'self' – where he could understand his connection to the universe and, crucially, know that he also held the universe within himself.

Today, this same path remains open to us all. Through Yoga and through Ayurveda, we may choose to live in a way that frees us from our self-imposed 'reality' which is, in fact, nothing other than our own thoughts projected onto any given moment in time.

Sattva: Pure Consciousness

In Ayurveda, we think about the 'four goals of life'. The three secondary goals are *kama, artha* and *dharma*. Kama is enjoyment. Artha is prosperity (the means to have what we need – clothing, food and shelter). Dharma is our career (rooted in purpose). Our primary goal is *moksha*, which is liberation. Moksha is freedom to express our needs, wishes and gifts fully, but to also feel free of obligation or worry – free of the trappings of life and the thoughts and judgements of others. Moksha can also be defined as inner peace, self-acceptance and knowledge. Through moksha we gain true intelligence – we see life for what it really is, and what we have been all along.

Sattva is the ultimate goal that rests above all four of these 'goals of life'. It is, in essence, freedom from all goals. A life in which we feel wholly, authentically liberated from sweating the small stuff – no ego, all essence. A life lived without walls.

The path that leads us there comes from Vedic science – a formalized system of knowledge taken from the Vedas (you'll learn about these in the Sattvic Resources section) and the sophisticated Indian civilization that gave us metaphysics and logic – placed into practical systems for living our most beautiful, awakened and fully realized lives.

The branches of Vedic science include Yoga and meditation, Ayurveda, Vedic astrology and *Vastu Shastra* (the science of 'environment' and architecture). In this book, we've chosen to focus on the science of sattva, as explained within Ayurveda and, to a slightly lesser degree, Yoga. We've done this consciously too. Not because Yoga's prevalence in the West is at fever pitch, while the living, breathing practice of Ayurveda often plays second fiddle, but because we want to lay the groundwork for sattvic living, which begins at a practical, physical level with the 'science of life'. This is Ayurveda every day.

Traditional Yoga, on the other hand, is more focused on the transcendent journey into spirit, and it's a deep, divine practice that was originally envisioned only for those who were strong, pure, clear and sattvic enough to transcend the physical body. Lay the groundwork first, is our feeling – something that Ayurveda does so beautifully, practically and transformatively.

During the reign of the British Raj in India (1858–1947), the schools of Ayurveda were forcibly closed down – Ayurvedic medicine was said to be backward, superstitious and founded neither on fact nor science (a cruel irony). This has done a great deal of deepest harm to us all. Our collective consciousness was wounded by such mistruth – with an ancient, hallowed, enlightened and awakened indigenous tradition of wisdom and healing banished from plain sight in the span of just a few brutal years.

A 5,000-year-old guiding, uniting, healing science was deemed 'quackery' by those who didn't understand it, feared it and therefore wanted to destroy it. That they didn't succeed reinforces that beautiful universal lesson – the truth is the truth, and it will rise. For if there's one law that can never be oppressed into oblivion, it is natural law.

Dr David Frawley, founder and director of the American Institute of Vedic Studies, has also noted that it was most likely at this point in history – when Ayurveda was discredited and expunged by the British, and schools of Ayurveda closed down across the Indian subcontinent – that Yoga began to exist apart from its Ayurvedic sister. Many millions of people readily adopted Yoga, but those practitioners who carried it to Western shores most often did so without any real link to, or knowledge of, its inherent bond with Ayurveda – both of which are rooted in the original Vedic texts.

THE GUNAS

Ayurveda tells us that there are three primal forces of nature, known as the *gunas*. The gunas are *tamas*, *rajas* and *sattva*. These three forces are inextricably connected – constantly interacting with, and impacting upon, one another; dominating or sinking into submission. Their dancing and interchange govern all of nature and creation. Each of the gunas has a place in all activity – cosmic, natural and human.

Tamas

This guna is heavy, static, destructive and negative. It's embodied; physical and material; an obstruction; the weight of the boulder as you press your whole body against it, and try to move it. It blocks you. *That* feeling is tamas. It's unconscious. It's darkness; the word is related to the Latin *temere*, meaning 'blindly'.

In people, tamas is ignorance, dullness, lack of sensitivity; the weight of habit, inertia. *Tamasic* people seek the material, to possess and to destroy. Their minds rest on physicality and the façade of a world perceived only through the senses – what Einstein referred to as the 'optical delusion', where we go through life experiencing our thoughts and feelings as separate from the thoughts and feelings of those around us.

Tamas is substance. It's finality, density and permanence. The tamasic mind is gloomy, lethargic, sad and repressed; it's morose: neither creative nor energized. While we must all shut off or close down at times, as we will see, it's not a mindset that brings joy or opportunity to us.

Rajas

This is the dynamism between the gunas. It's action, activity and movement, change and disruption; impetus, aggression and expansion. Rajas is inherently unstable. It's flux, always transition, never settling or achieving equilibrium. It's the energy that brings us dawn and dusk, rise and fall, the passing into and out of the day. It's the stone thrown at the still lake that sets off a concentric pulse of ripples. Rajas is the swing between love and hate or attraction and repulsion.

We modern humans have become increasingly *rajasic*. We dream, motivate, propel. We are rushing, juggling, panicking – ever between things, places, feelings. Our cultural norms have us all in 'red shoes': our lives are frenetic, the candle of our mind always weathered; they are increasingly, mercilessly, stimulated so must dance and dance, but have largely forgotten stillness. Rajas is doing, thinking, moving. It's not, though, being.

Sattva

Sattva is light, love and consciousness. It's unifying and harmonizing; purity and clarity; peace and serenity; pure awareness and being. Daylight.

SATTVA

Sattva is *life*. A sattvic human seeks truth – the realization of self over physicality; moderation and higher experience over material gain and possession. Such a person is peaceful, aware, empathetic and gentle; they tend towards those things we characterize as 'good' and 'noble'.

A rajasic person may be materially 'rich' but feel poor and dissatisfied. A sattvic person will feel rich in all circumstances, irrespective of material wealth, and with good reason – they have endless gratitude for life itself. Sattva is also balancing, and it harmonizes the positive of rajas with the negative of tamas.

The gunas are rarely to be found in their pure form. Equally, people are not purely sattvic, rajasic or tamasic, but always a combination of the three that's constantly changing. Rajas moves us towards either sattva or tamas. We have two rajasic forces: the higher, heading towards sattva, and the lower, which takes us to tamas. Through our practices and our choices we may cultivate a sort of polarization towards ever-greater sattva. This is the naturally awakening and elevating path of both Yoga and Ayurveda.

Intention, and small, sattvic choices are essential here. Rajas is important: we must move, get up and get on; and crucially, we must adjust. But we can choose sattvic movement – conducting ourselves well and kindly as we move through our lives. And while tamas allows us to be grounded, and necessarily lost in sleep each night, sattvic inertia provides healing, sound sleep, and beyond that, the deepest rest and renewal of Vedic meditation (you'll learn about this later in the book).

LIVING A SATTVIC LIFE

When we adopt a sattvic mindset and way of living, life itself – the literal 'things' that make up the 'day' – may not change, but the way it feels will be completely transformed. We will continue to wake, eat breakfast and go to work. There will still be challenges aplenty, but we can choose to react to them in a panicked, impatient, frustrated way, or we can approach the highs and lows with equanimity, perspective and patience – the essence of sattva.

We have two young children, numerous 'jobs' and live in a little house without home help or childcare, so we say this from not just the heart, but our pragmatists' heads too. With so much to do, we've made fundamental adjustments to our priorities that have brought with them greater peace of mind, and living is now richer and easier in its flow – the hours not stretched but aligned. This is a change in rhythm more than substance, and it's all the more profound for it.

Sattva is not about creating a 'perfect life' – nobody has that power. It doesn't ask that each morning begins with birdsong and an hour spent smelling the roses (but, if you can rise before or alongside the sun, and find a few moments to watch it climb the horizon – oh yes, sattva will abound there, and be carried within you as you enter your day).

We always have the power to cultivate a 'self' that can react and respond to challenge in a positive way. Sattva guides us, always, closer to our truest and most authentic self. When we're able to step back from the confusion, mixed messaging, monkey mind and limiting beliefs we have about ourselves and the world we live in, and really *feel* our way into life instead, we begin to understand what makes us thrive – who we are, at the very core of our beings; what our essence is all about, when it's removed from the overbearing voice of our ego.

We make better, kinder decisions. We walk in line with our belief systems (because we're finally able to tap into our authentic purpose) and all that weight of unnecessary worry, overthinking and self-sabotage just falls completely away.

HOW THIS BOOK WORKS

There's a reason this book contains seven chapters. Within the limits of page count and printing and portability, we've chosen to celebrate the very essence of sattva in the simplest possible ways – as simple as the simplest things in life (which, as we know right down to the heartstrings, are simply the best things of all).

While reading this book, we hope that you'll see, feel and experience the way that it moves through layers of the self – from the grounded and rooted first chapter, which talks about our place on this beautiful Earth, to the seventh chapter, which celebrates our innate ability to meditate our way to the higher planes of consciousness that are our natural birthright. The book also implicitly mirrors the energies and forces that preside within each of the body's seven chakras (energy centres) from root to crown – moving from Earth-born, childhood and ancestral ties to the highest, freest, most awakened essence of our being.

The experience of this book very consciously reflects that of the Vedic sages of old, who knew that for anyone to meditate successfully and shed unnecessary, weighty, painful layers of self-limit, greed, grief, regret, ill-mind and health, they first had to prepare the terrain. Your terrain is not just your body: it's the whole of your life – from the thoughts you choose to entertain to the company you like to keep, the energy of your environment and the ritual and rhythm of the every day.

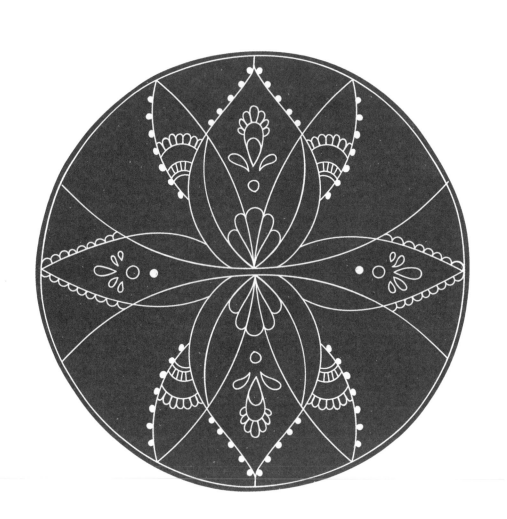

CHAPTER 1

UNITY

'Of a certainty, the man who can see all creatures in himself, himself in all creatures, knows no sorrow.'

THE ISHA UPANISHAD

W E BELIEVE THAT LIFE CAN BE HUGELY ENRICHED when we feel united and connected to all around us – when we step back and realize that nothing exists in isolation, including ourselves. Ayurveda provides an integrated holistic approach to living and wellbeing which understands that every aspect of a person's lifestyle impacts upon all other aspects and all other lives.

We may suspect that we're a single thread in a greater tapestry, but when we seek to remove ourselves, we find that we're intricately bound with every other thread, each one of us an equally essential part of the big 'picture'. In this chapter we explore the transformative potential for profound unity – remembering our place amongst, not apart from, all life – and present a view of our world as a cohesive whole, formed of the interplay between universal consciousness and energy: the foundations of Vedic understanding.

LIVING HOLISTICALLY

Gravitating from an 'ordinary life' – one where you get knocked sideways and buried under even the smallest problem or worry – to a life where you transcend the little things and find your own 'big picture', involves taking a journey. For the Vedic sages, it began with Ayurveda.

The word Ayurveda means 'the knowledge of life' – *ayu* means life and *veda* means science, knowledge and wisdom. Ayurveda provides the clearest possible road map – not to some distant, dreamed-of pinnacle of optimal health and a perfect life, but back to your own birthright: vitality, joy, bliss.

As the sages believed that the full, unified practice of Yoga and meditation must *begin* by grounding ourselves in the holistically supportive lifestyle, embodied by Ayurveda, we can see how a lot of us in the West have these things backwards.

Yoga – the spiritual practice that takes us to self-actualization – was a final destination; a journey to highest consciousness. While they overlap, Ayurveda is something more down-to-earth than Yoga – the path to self-healing that strengthens, purifies and balances the many aspects of body and mind so that we may graduate onwards to a successful, unified Yoga practice. Ayurveda and Yoga are Vedic siblings who play most beautifully *together*.

As you'll discover in this book, there's comprehensive Ayurvedic advice available for every imaginable facet of our lives – from oral hygiene to sexual activity; from digestion to sleep; and from mental disorder to chronic constipation. In Ayurveda and Yoga, sattva is celebrated as the highest energy – not as something to attain to, which is lofty, far-fetched and impossibly aspirational, but the opposite: as something that's our natural path. Sattva is most keenly felt, within the depths of our being, when we're as close as we can be to nature – our own, and that of the world all around us.

We're approaching a new Galileo moment; a remembering of our wholeness. It will be akin to looking back as we do today and wondering how our ancestors ever believed the world was flat or the Earth was the still centre of the universe around which everything moves.

That last example, the font of Galileo's heresy when he expressed the Copernican view that the sun, rather than the Earth, is central to the solar system, speaks to an egoistic tendency we have as humans – the great *humanist* religion – to set ourselves apart from everything else in creation and assume that we are, literally, the centre of the universe. We do this on an individual level too. We prioritize our needs over those of others, and feel justified in manipulating and mastering other species and natural beings.

The Truth and Miracle of Life

The searching of cosmologists, physicists and mathematicians for an elegant equation or grand unified theory that will encapsulate all natural law, account for all universal forces and explain exactly what will happen in the future, has found us here, somewhere in one of 10^{500} universes, with 11 dimensions (at last count) and within which everything that could have happened, has indeed happened. Where Schrödinger's cat is both alive and dead. Or perhaps we're somewhere else entirely. We spiral through time and space and litter it with stories and events that are happening still. Only left behind.

The world doesn't become less miraculous the more we understand of it. Quite the opposite. Our universe is a vast field, a playground of infinite excitation, resonance and interaction. Behind the physical phenomena we experience through our senses is a profound unity – the creative energy and consciousness that all forces, objects, elements, stars, butterflies, teaspoons and we ourselves, fundamentally are.

This isn't to say that our world is one of illusion. It's a vehicle of miracles, of unimaginable expression – at once personal and shared by all; the most vivid and vital of action paintings. And behind it all, as both the Vedas and Schrödinger have told us: ALL IS ONE.

We've heard it said that philosophy is dead. This may be true when it comes to philosophy drawn from the intellect, but we believe that there are answers to be gained from the whole act of *being*; from locating that self that is essence and pure awareness. It's because that self, that highest consciousness, is the very same one that's shared by everyone and everything. It holds all the answers about who we are. We would modify the philosopher Rene Descartes' dictum '*I think, therefore I am*' to simply: '*I am, but not so much when I am thinking.*'

This understanding has taken many forms in recent years and pervades many a self-help and self-care manual and manifesto. It's the essence of mindfulness and of witnessing; and the way of classical Yoga and meditation in all its forms. It lives in all those books about knitting, spoon-carving or building wood fires; where action emanates from the body and thought is simply allowed to flow – not forced or suppressed.

We would distil this instinct further to the simple Sanskrit mantra *So ham* (pronounced so hum), which means *I am that*. 'I am' refers to individual consciousness; 'that' to universal consciousness. Both of these elements are one. Each of us is 'that'.

We're all precious and wondrous and extraordinary – in the same way that every other living thing is too – because there is no distinction to be made.

ONE IS ALL. And there are no exceptions.

FROM THE GROUND UP

Let's begin with our roots. Human beings have become increasingly isolated. There was a time when we were an inextricable part of the world, when nature's rhythms were our own. Our rise from mere monkey status to the top of the food chain was too speedy, propelled inordinately by our harnessing of fire and tools; through cooking and filling sails with the elements to cross the seas.

These were cheaty factors in the context of evolution: previously unavailable to any of the world's creatures and, as such, leaving the natural world with no time to evolve so that it could accommodate an explosion in the human population. Crucially, *we* didn't have time to adjust either – to evolve ways to accept and assimilate our status – so rapidly did we shoot to dominance.

The dawn of agriculture – generally placed around 12,000 years ago – added to the hierarchical and competitive modes of living that have come to define our modern age. Through cultivation, and domesticating, mastering and controlling animals, we set ourselves apart from the whole. We decided that our station is to hover a little above the rest. We also began to feel more frightened – tied to the places we'd started to cultivate – and found far less time in which to relax and commune. The short chapter of violence, competition and extraction that has followed shows how we increasingly set ourselves apart from one another too, and how that has damaged the human psyche and the planet we call home.

The gift that truly distinguished we *homo sapiens* from the other human species with whom we once shared the planet was our storytelling. We didn't have the largest brains, nor were we the strongest physically, but the sweeping narratives we were able to conjure proved more powerful than these factors. They allowed us to unite on unprecedented levels. Spiritual beliefs, myth and parable brought us together. This is incredibly interesting when viewed alongside our modern times, the stories we're now telling, and what these say about the levels of consciousness in which we're living.

The hunter-gatherers and pre-agricultural tribes still in existence today (at least, those that we're still able to observe directly) tell stories of forest spirits and direct communion with their environments. They warn against competition, and assuming higher station or leadership, and have developed spiritual practices both to protect their open, egalitarian social structures and to deepen their connection to the natural surrounds that sustain and protect them. These stories and practices allow them to attain levels of consciousness where this subtle osmosis of information can be directly perceived – where everything is a whole of which they are simply a part.

The *truth* of these stories is energetic, experiential and practical rather than literal. It reflects what's experienced, intuited and lived. It's felt or imparted rather than reasoned or intellectualized.

We've realized that, here in our modern settings, amongst our modern systems and pursuits, the most ancient and profound of balances is off. Something extremely powerful is lacking. This something is sattva.

A UNIFIED SYSTEM OF HEALING

To think of ourselves as *whole* can be hard. We so often feel fragmented and divided – between 10 different tasks and a mile of to-dos – personally and societally. Ayurveda presents a very different way of thinking about our *self*. The self is a concept unrelated to the physical body – it transcends it. It's pure consciousness: *being* rather than doing. Our being unites us all: an infinite vista of flickering wicks lit from the same fire.

As we've already touched upon, from the fundamental understanding that we're reflections of, and inseparable from, nature and the universe,

Vedic sages and seers have been busy for millennia observing, recounting and chronicling the diverse ways in which we may live in harmony with all the forces, energies and resonances of the wider world.

In meditation and spiritual practices they found the stems and branches of Yoga, which (you may have noticed) has retained a certain appeal and pervaded the modern West. Ayurveda, too, arose from Vedic teachings over 5,000 years ago as a kind of sub-Veda (*upaveda*) and has lost no relevance, in spite of brutal colonial oppression and the proliferation of modern medicine.

Yoga is literally 'union': the 'yoking', or drawing together, of forces under practice and discipline towards self-realization. Our modern, Western, tendency, however, has often been to un-yoke it. *Asana*, the posture and movement of Yoga, is but one aspect of it, and a lower one when held against elements such as *bhakti* or *jnana* – the Yogas of devotion and knowledge, or the *yamas* and *niyamas*, which govern ethics and integrity: the first two 'limbs' of the eight Yoga sutras imagined by the sage Patanjali.

Ayurveda is the most unified of healing systems. Where allopathy is treatment using opposites and homeopathy is treatment using similars, Ayurveda incorporates both and is open to an incredibly broad and complex therapeutic landscape. Its knowledge base is simply incredible, and for the most part, incredibly simple. It taps us back into the thing that we once all relied upon for survival: our instincts (in which we find the ancestral knowledge we've stored), intuition and common sense.

Ayurveda is integrated healing that sees the interconnectedness of body, mind and spirit; which treats and anticipates according to the individuality of every person, their situation, lifestyle and environment. It spans every aspect of living, and emphasizes self-knowledge and lifestyle tweaks towards the prevention of ill health in the first place, and at its root cause – rather than a curative or reactive treatment of symptoms.

In Ayurveda we have a complete lifestyle prescription that invites us to do what already comes naturally. To wake with the sun, cast light into the dark and melt away coldness with soul-satiating warmth. We're born knowing how to thrive – sleeping, feeding, eliminating, nuzzling – no one teaches us these things.

The body and mind heal by themselves when they are allowed to. Ayurveda is a science that reunites every single thing that makes us *us*, and that touches us too. Our bodies, our minds, our spirits, our energy, our communities and our world: Ayurveda understands that none of these exists independently, and each affects and is affected by the actions and reactions that make up our lifestyles. Everything is profoundly interconnected and bound in delicate relativity.

All That You Need, You Already Are

The very idea of a *lifestyle* is a drawing together of many things. *Life* is the thing that we have and share. With *style* comes aspiration. A lifestyle book will sit on the lifestyle shelf, where we may leaf through many different lifestyles belonging to many different people. Selecting one, you can seek to mould the life you already have, so that it looks a bit more like someone else's.

A lifestyle book is something to be sold. So, too, is the lifestyle and the image of the person living it. Often though, we try on this image and realize that it's not our own. We count our change and return to the lifestyle shelf, still seeking, still incomplete.

Ayurveda understands that there's a still, serene lake inside each of us, of unimaginable depth. What we need is innate, natural, powerful and *already within us*. When we start on a new path, we often begin by considering each step; simply and consciously putting one foot in front of the other. We may at times pause, look over our shoulder or backtrack a little but, as we continue, the walk becomes increasingly effortless as the need to consider or compare falls away and a deeper intelligence – our innate wisdom – is awakened.

We begin to realize that the aspirational end point we set out envisioning – all of those goals we set and signposts we sought – are actually unnecessary. The most meaningful route to a 'lifestyle' that is ours, and ours alone, is revealed by the path itself and the qualities of consciousness it opens up to us.

With all new beginnings, there's a conscious choice to be made. Like a rolled-up carpet on a gentle hill, there's a little impetus required to set it unfolding. After a while though, it's easy – the carpet unfurls without effort or exertion, and the way becomes so obvious as to be instinctive. Just like breathing.

Importantly, while we can access shelves and stores and databases stacked high with myriad means by which to bring greater wellness to our existing 'lifestyles', our lives will also naturally evolve with our consciousness. Where higher consciousness goes, the stuff of our lives will follow. You may be surprised as to where.

THE RISE IN SATTVA

Socially, culturally, familially, we're often heavily conditioned to seek out particular modes of success and fulfilment. These tend to be rooted in transient touchlines – physical things that we can hold, drive and possess. They, too, are rooted in our movement: our need to grind, work, graft, earn, conquer and thereby secure all the 'stuff' of the 'happy ending'.

Happiness and awareness in a purer sense are often lost to this conditioning, or sacrificed on the altar of 'growth' – we live and sweat the small stuff, unrelentingly. Entire years are lost to heightened stress, overwork, lack of sleep, insufficient time… the extra hours put in to achieve an upgraded lifestyle or significant pay rise eclipsing any sense of how we may, ourselves, truly rise. How we may, in fact, really *live* the lives that we work so incredibly hard to fund. How we may begin to prioritize other things, instead – the joy and magic of the moment; of simple pleasure and experience; or, you know, just being.

As we'll explore later, Ayurveda knows that pain doesn't bring gain. You're hurting yourself to effect a particular change in your physical being – but what about your neglected spirit? Your fractious mind, your hungry soul? Feed your spirit, nourish your soul, heal your mind and understand that these aren't separate entities but parts of a whole – each element exchanging, facilitating, dancing with the others – and your body and soul and mind will bloom and flourish and reflect all of your sattva right back at you.

PRANAYAMA FOR UNITY – UNIFIED BREATH

The word *pranayama* is derived from the Sanskrit *prana*, meaning 'life force' or 'vital energy', and *ayama*, meaning 'extension'. Pranayama is the bringing of conscious awareness to the breath through specific techniques and exercises. There are many types of pranayama – some of which can be found in this book – and each creates a different sensation and feeling of balance. Depending on the type being practiced, pranayama might energize us or cool us down, encourage deeper sleep or dispel anxiety.

Yogic sectional breathing, or *dirgha pranayama*, promotes awareness of the different ways in which we breathe, and how bringing unity and awareness to our breath can lead to deep and lasting calm. A complete yogic breath utilizes all three chambers of the lungs, from the abdomen through the thorax and clavicle and back again, so it's also known as a three-part breath. Practising each part helps us to assimilate breathing more fully into our daily lives. In turn, our lungs experience improved release of toxins, our blood is better oxygenated and our bodies and minds are more relaxed and better fed.

Practise the first three stages below for five breaths each, and be aware of the difference and any changes in sensation:

1. Begin with abdominal breathing. Sit upright in a relaxed position and hold your right palm to your abdomen. As you inhale, slowly push out your abdomen and then draw it inwards as you exhale. Keep your inhalation and exhalation long, slow and equal.

2. Next, expand your chest as you inhale, maintaining the same length and balance of breath. As you exhale, feel your chest and ribcage contract.

3. Now hold your hands to the back of your shoulders. As you inhale, bring your elbows close to one another. As you exhale, move them away from one another, maintaining your slow, regular breathing.

4. Now practise complete yogic breathing. This is a combination of all three of the stages above. As you inhale, inflate your abdomen, expand upwards into your chest and further into your shoulders. As you exhale, allow all three chambers to empty slowly – contract the shoulders, then the chest and then the abdomen.

This is what we mean when we talk about 'breathing deeply'. It doesn't refer to the force of your breath, but rather to the space created through which your breath may flow. Keep your posture upright and shoulders raised and breathe through all three chambers. Yogic sectional breathing can be practiced anywhere at any time and will bring immediate calm and greater clarity.

REUNITE WITH YOUR INNER KNOWING

There's a great ocean of joy and knowing all around us, and we're often frightened to swim in it, lest the plug be unexpectedly pulled. Nevertheless, this is the swim we're offering in this book. While there's a growing understanding of Ayurveda in the West, and we're beginning to see the relevance for our times in its poetic, kind and expansive wisdom, what we might call its spiritual side is often lost to its more physical truths.

Many modern approaches to Ayurveda focus on two things: the 'body type' (a simplification of the primary forces within our body, called the *doshas*; you'll learn more about these in Chapter 2) and the foods we should then eat in order to balance that body type. There's huge merit and efficacy in this; however, it's just one tiny part of the whole, because our body is just one tiny part of our self.

While knowing our dosha gives us valuable knowledge of our individual, inbuilt tendencies, it's important to understand that our 'actual' balance may be quite different at any given time, shifting as it must with the seasons, weather and time of day, as well as our diet, environment, activities, habits and sleeping patterns.

We believe that it's really important to see Ayurveda in its wider, more unified context – including its place amongst the Vedas, with particular emphasis on its sister science, Yoga. As much as Ayurveda is a unified system of medicine, it's also a manual by which we can begin to decipher the language of nature – our very own nature and constitution, personality and proclivities, as much as the world of nature that surrounds us (but which, with the busy-ness of modern life, we can sometimes half-forget about).

We, ourselves, make up the ever-shifting *life* that we live, as much as our ebbing and flowing seas, cycling moon, rising and setting sun and ever-changing seasons. This is our every thing and our every day (even if our job keeps us in a climate-controlled cubicle for most of the year).

When we move away from nature, we lose our way. When we sit up late, working long past sunset, and then pass out from exhaustion and slumber into the afternoon; when we charge up our phones and laptops so we can keep on keeping on, long after our own internal batteries have gone entirely flat; when we attempt to continue conversations with our cherished loved ones while frantically replying to a dozen urgent emails: with one eye on each and our hearts in none, we have, indeed, lost our way.

We have, both of us, done all of the above, many times over, and each and every time, it harmed us, in ways big and small... until we got to a point when we'd really just had enough. *Stop looking for happiness in the place where you lost it* is one of our favourite mottos. In Ayurveda, that place is the point where you remove yourself from nature. When you decide that you can outsmart nature – with energizing drinks or pills, perhaps, or numbing painkillers, or simply by pushing things down so very far that you'll never have to look at them in the light of day again.

THE PATH OF SATTVA

The only way – and it's the Vedic way – to unite your self with your very best health, is to return to your natural instincts, your intuition, your needs, your cycles, your inner wisdom, and to embody them all, unapologetically, lovingly and wholly. To go slowly and gently enough that you can begin to listen, properly, to what it is that you really need, and to be loving and generous enough with your self to be able to offer it up, as painlessly and instinctively as breathing, each and every time.

Back to our self, and reconnected to our inner sattva, we may once again awaken our own innate powers of healing and incredible reservoirs of energy, love and compassion; or luxuriate in our serene inner pools of calm without simply substituting modern medicines for exotic Himalayan plants, many of which are increasingly endangered.

As we'll discuss in Chapter 6, diet is important under Ayurveda, but *food* is understood as a greater unity: all that we take in from the world around us – what we eat, breathe, imbibe and absorb through impressions, images and our associations. It's also the ways in which we take on these things, the spirit in which they are received and the extent to which we're prepared for them.

Are we grabbing and running and inhaling our food, or are we slowing, creating, opening up and properly receiving it, instead? Are we choosing to eat food that comes from unknown places, filled with mysterious things and tasting of nothing much at all? Or are we consciously choosing nourishment – eating with reverence and wholehearted enjoyment; the spirit and body connected as we do so?

The everyday experience can be bitty and discordant. It can also be a beautiful dance: exultant and harmonious. The choice, truly, is yours. We don't need to overhaul our lifestyles, only invite more sattva into our increasingly buffeted, darting and material mind. And as we begin to do so, we may find that we *want* to overhaul – as we appreciate the increasing symbiosis and harmonizing of our bodies and brains. Through simple, sattvic steps, we can change the angle at which we enter the world and the glass through which we view it.

We *homo sapiens* have the potential for incredible unity. Through our storytelling and our spirituality we became the most unified of primates. Today, we're moving steadily towards a single, global human society (though it may be one that's destructive and egotistical enough to be doomed – such is often the plotting of our modern stories).

We believe, however, that our storytelling can inspire a greater unity still – one that encompasses the whole: of nature and humanity. We believe that through embarking on the path of sattva, we may approach and tap into the most expansive and timeless harmonies: those of highest consciousness and the very essence of being. Our stories can be incredibly powerful.

We begin with a deep breath, and a little of our own story.

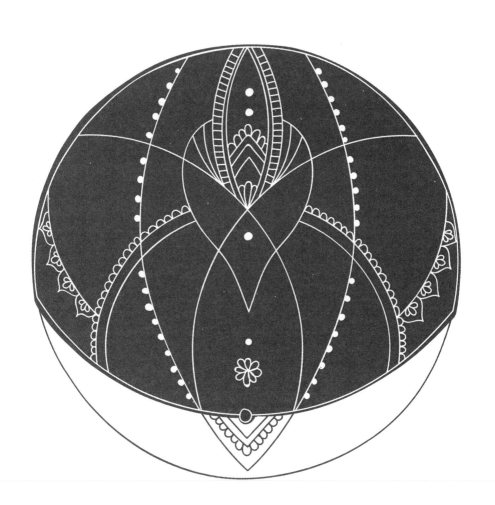

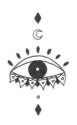

CHAPTER 2

HARMONY

*'We know that every particle in the physical universe
takes its characteristics from the pitch and pattern
and overtones of its particular frequencies, its
singing. Before we make music, music makes us.'*

JOACHIM-ERNST BERENDT, *THE WORLD IS SOUND*

THERE IS BOTH FREEDOM AND COMFORT to be found in aligning our lifestyles more closely with the wider world and the rhythms of nature. In this chapter we shed light on our own harmonic potential – looking at the ways we can tune in to and honour each of nature's elements, qualities and forces, as well as the natural and celestial cycles that reflect and illuminate our own. We'll explain how the sun, moon and wind impact upon the daily, monthly and seasonal ordering of our energies, and explore simple, enjoyable ways to bring increased harmony to our homes and routines.

OUR SATTVA STORY

Spiritual awakenings come with different levels of urgency. If we're lucky it will be like the emerging brightness on a Sunday – the sharpening glister of birdsong gently calling us into newness and awareness, deliciously slowly and with perfect ease, like the sun or the rise of a good loaf. Sometimes we're jolted awake. Things happen suddenly and painfully to reveal the extent to which we've drifted from spiritual health – or to remind us that our spirit was ever even there in the first place.

We deepened our interest in Ayurveda ten years ago, shortly after conceiving our first child. We'd long leaned towards conscious living; we tried to tie ourselves more profoundly to the natural world and to be responsible global citizens through actions which, while helpful and important in our modern context, can also seem a little abstract, striking somewhere shy of the heart of the matter.

We busied ourselves with sourcing organic, fair-trade food, coffee and clothing; buying household products and cosmetics without mineral oils or uncertified palm oils; with offsetting our paper and vapour trails. We were, back then, without even discussing it, walking back home to nature, baby step by baby step.

We learned – as Ayurveda has always known – that the world we live in closely mirrors our own selves. The universe is the macrocosm, the human 'self' the microcosm. And because we're indivisible, whenever we seek to remove ourselves from nature – and our *own* nature: our calling, our purpose, our dharma – we feel deeply sad, isolated, increasingly desperate.

We believe that almost everybody will relate to that feeling of having to swim against the self – when we ignore our gut instincts and push ourselves into situations where we feel blocked; or when we awake in cold, uninviting darkness and stay plugged-in long after dusk.

In our home the windows were always closed against the dust, drone and blether of the road; the blinds against the blinking lights. The weather, the seasons, the celestial cycles were all just things going on outside that we might briefly enter on the walk to the bus stop or Tube station. Like so many, we were detached from nature and struggling to explain, quantify or justify the isolation, unhappiness and anxiety we felt. Paul broke down entirely. Work that was at first rewarding became heartbreaking and almost impossible. The simplest things became difficult – sleeping, waking, eating, talking. The lights went out for a time. Around us, too, micro mirrored macro. Herbs struggled in pots on the little balcony overlooking the busy, polluted, ill-tempered road below – our daily soil was too poor to support us. We'd chosen the buzz of the city; access to work opportunities that didn't exist outside; snippets of community found in passing, in work colleagues and in our phones.

There was a reason why we felt drawn, almost daily, to the long walk that took us into the heart of London's Greenwich Park, where we'd sit surrounded by old cedars and sweet chestnuts and never want to leave. We felt at ease there – as we all do in our parks and gardens, forests and fields, where sattva abounds.

We fought a losing battle for peace with the cortisol flooding our system with every siren, almost here, almost gone; each adrenalized workday and impatient traffic at all hours. The reasons for the darkest of times can be incredibly elusive, contained as they often are in shadowy corners of our selves. Like everybody else, we were always logged-on. Our working situations rendered us unable to be unavailable (or so we told ourselves); while we became increasingly so to the world outside of work.

There's a loneliness to modern urban living and our social mobility. While we exist quite apart from all other species (and increasingly so from one another and often from all meaningful sense of community), we're ostensibly more connected than ever. While physically apart we're not allowed that exquisite experience of missing someone, or even leaving someone behind. We carry one another in our pockets: our families and friends in this hemisphere or the other. But our communion is a strange and filtered interface, where we fill in the blanks between the characters pinged around the world, and forgotten people we knew at school allow us access to their triumphs and breakfast.

Each affirmation we receive in this way, each alert telling us that our updates are approved of, brings an unsustainable spike in our dopamine levels, the likes of which our ancestors could never have imagined. Chemically, these encounters can be more interesting, more dramatic, than our 'real-life' interactions, and we become lost in them, along with everybody else in our train carriage (which now has decent Wi-Fi, to boot).

The same is true of much processed food and the to-and-fro between *wanting* and *acquiring*. A lot of undue rising and dipping that, in evolutionary terms, we've only recently had to contend with and are not equipped to handle well. Where our ancestors entered 'fight-or-flight' mode, shutting down all but the most vital human functions in order to send a flood of energy towards fleeing across the savannah or doing battle with immediate threats to their lives, we do the same at the cancellation of a train, a hard word from a work colleague or our misplaced keys; at the drop of a hat.

Such emergency functions, now integrated incongruously into our day-to-day lifestyles, are what we call stress. At the end of the day, and the beginning, we were just two people in a box on the high road, overly wired and increasingly tired, self-medicating these unquantified factors and travelling to work in a bubble.

Reconnecting Through Nature

This is *real life*, depending on who you're talking to: a little disharmony, but nothing wrong. Unable to get our slow, graceful rise off the ground, we awoke instead with a bump. While preparing for our baby's arrival, we were drawn to one book – Dr Gowri Motha's *The Gentle Birth Method* – the presiding wisdom of which was rooted in Ayurveda.

This beautiful, intuitive, preparative approach jogged our memories of the snatches of Vedic and yogic practice we'd experienced; at once spiritual and immensely practical. It raised intoxicating ghosts of travel in India – the kind with backpacks on shoestrings and dog-eared copies of the *Bhagavad Gita* and Gandhi's *Experiments with Truth*.

The miracle of our first baby – that most fundamental magic – our world suddenly her world, her world newly ours, set us dreaming as we held her in a single palm, and we began to immerse ourselves in Ayurveda once more. Returning to Vedic wisdom helped us to better understand our relationships with nature and with the modern world.

As the Himalayan sages gleaned, thousands of years before the birth of Christ, the external world closely mirrors our own selves. There's a unity and beautiful harmony to all of existence that runs converse to much of our modern context. When we live apart from nature, or any overarching sense of a connected whole, our days, actions, health and convictions can easily seem separate.

Other people, other species, other places – all is division; painful and isolating. The human diversity that we loved and celebrated in our city of London, which excited and nourished us so hugely, was undercut on the one hand by the accompanying social and institutional inequalities, and on the other by the lack of diversity that wasn't human.

Naturally, kindly, our baby daughter led us away from the city to the village; to a friendly terrace and a little cottage framed and flanked by woodland. A small community opened up to us, along with each of the seasons, the night sky and layer upon layer of life. Each spoke harmony.

The winter that had previously meant bigger coats and darker mornings became something more expansive: a shiver through the landscape; fine wood vapour from the village chimneys; the brittle shimmer to the grass underfoot that lights each tread. Each shift brought changes that our urban awareness had been unable to perceive – the introspection of autumn; the digestion and assimilation in the cold earth of winter; the new expression and cleansing of spring and the sheer, raucous vibrancy of summer.

We began to grow food and flowers, which connected us further to the seasons, the earth and the elements. We began to feel quieted and somehow held. A place in these more natural environments seemed to open up much larger, more profound vistas of consciousness. We'd found our home in the big picture – one that made sense, one that put a lot of the petty stuff into perspective, at last.

The moon, now much more visible, looming over the ancient conifers that hide our cottage from the road, also felt more present, more relevant. We felt more involved in her cycling – thoughtful and quieter when she began to wane; more determined and replete in her fullness.

We became aware of something that we'd rarely felt since childhood – nature's ever-shifting, adjusting and balancing *rta*: its rhythm. There are entire, subtle symphonies of sound in our natural world – birdsong and bee hum – that we'd forgotten. We felt, so very keenly, how we'd allowed our lives to become so disconnected from these subtleties as to become discordant. While nature shifted key, innumerable times each and every day, we'd spent years missing it all. Summer seemed to disappear overnight and plunge us into the shock of winter without so much as a transitioning moment – from over-hot and red and frantic, to mulch and sludge, bitter and hard on the chest.

The life we'd chosen had no harmony, and no rhythm. What we had, really, was a full calendar year of white noise – filtered, centrally heated and air-conditioned. We ate the same stuff, day in day out; we walked the same road, caught the same train, found the same seat and forgot to stare out of the window at all.

Today, we're a family of four and are busier than ever; we're of modest means and poor on time, yet we feel incongruously that the pressure is off. With more subtlety and less volume, our shoulders dropped and the anxiety ebbed. Ayurveda now makes experiential sense. At its root it understands, as many ancient systems did, that we *are* nature. Dis-ease and ill health is simply the distance we fly from Mother Nature and her embracing, protecting and healing principles. And, for us, living what we've lived, and feeling what we've felt, we know that even one step removed is a step too far.

A NEW DAY – THE VEDIC WAY

For a long time, we had no sense of how to live life in rhythm with nature – neither our own nor that of the cycling world around us. We stayed up long past 11 p.m. and worked/played into the wee hours; commuting on those strip-lit trains before sunrise and after sunset with little sense of where we were. And while the day's work must still be done, and sometimes natural laws are broken in the process, we know, most keenly, that we feel our best when we rise with the sun, and settle to sleep before we're tempted by that 'second wind' of doing.

That early scratch of the throat, tightness of the shoulders, throb in the back of the head – we must pay attention to it. That heaviness of the eyelids, slowing of speech, dullness of the mind – we must pay attention to that too. These are signals from the body that we're fighting the day's natural energy, and are out of harmony, not just with our self, but our nature.

Today we can feel the shifting energies of the gunas, the primal energies of nature (rajas, tamas and sattva) in the course of a single day. Sunshine, with its essential life-giving light and luminosity, embodies sattva. The dark, heavy, swaddling blanket of night-time, and semiconsciousness in sleep, is tamas. And as we shift from sunrise into the day, and sunset into the night, we find ourselves living with the energy of rajas, which moves us between sattva and tamas.

The effect upon our minds, though, at sunrise and sunset, can feel very different. When rajas moves us into sattva – in that time before the sun comes to rise, with all the promise of a new day and a fresh start – our minds tend to be light, free and positive; this is purposeful, optimistic and motivated rajas in action.

When, instead, rajas moves us from the energy of the day into the darkness of night – in that time before the sun prepares to set – our minds can move towards anxiety, self-doubt and overthinking. This is rajas that arises from the restless mind – a place where the fears creep in, thick and fast.

Natural Vedic Rhythms

These shifts in energy, from morning to evening, occur every day. Centuries before scientific studies revealed the body's biological clocks, its circadian rhythms and chronotypes, Ayurveda had already witnessed how the body ebbs and flows throughout the course of a single 24-hour cycle. If we force ourselves to stay awake, alert and plugged in far longer than nature ever intended for us, we'll feel that discordancy soon enough – just as ignoring the harmony between day and night can quickly lead us to a world where all is topsy-turvy.

Becoming more aware of the day's natural rhythm is an empowering thing. In the West, we often view a dip in energy as some sort of failing. We're sat at a desk, with no fresh air and little movement, for upwards of an hour, and then wonder why our brains run dry. We're not made to be constant; we're creatures who thrive on natural fluctuations and adjustments, growth and responsiveness.

Ayurveda explains the day's changing rhythms in a way that illuminates the body's natural proclivities – empowering us to work alongside them rather than against them, and making us mindful of overexerting, forcing or pushing ourselves. Now, instead of reaching for an energizing boost of caffeine or sugar mid-afternoon, we both know that mid-afternoon isn't meant to be a time of sustained doing.

A naturally airier energy pervades after lunchtime, which makes us feel less tethered to our work and purpose. It's harder, therefore, to carry on with sedentary pursuits – the mind is naturally flightier, so this energy is naturally conducive to a brainstorming stroll, some outdoor journalling, or simply meditating in a way that quells the overactive mind while still encouraging creativity. The way we build our days has started to nod, ever more truthfully, to the very nature at play within the day itself.

The Five Great Elements

Nature is full of shifting rhythms and cycles, energies and forces, and it can be difficult to think about them in isolation. That's because they aren't literally graspable – no one can hold the wind or cut a slice of space to display on the shelf.

In Ayurveda, all that exists is manifested from the Five Great Elements (*Pancha Mahabhutas*), which are ether (or space), air, fire, water and earth. These five elements are the essential building blocks of the entire universe and everything within it, and Ayurveda looks at how these elements manifest not just in the world around us, but within us too. Each of these elements also relates to one of the five senses – and it's through this sense that we come to understand the element as it appears in the world around us.

The elements, and the primal energies of sattva, rajas and tamas, are not finite or static. This makes sense because no living thing is ever still or unchanging.

◊ **Ether (or space)** is pure sattva, and the four elements beneath ether are like rungs of a ladder that eventually lead us there. Ether is the element that goes beyond the physical; it cannot be contained or quantified – it's the primal energy of pure consciousness. Ether relates to our sense of sound, and we tune in to the 'space' around us through our ears.

◊ **The air** around us is always in motion – this is the primal energy of change and propulsion: rajas. Air is related to our sense of touch, and we're made aware of this element via our skin.

◊ **Fire** is both sattvic in its ability to illuminate and cast light into darkness, and rajasic, because it's heating, catalysing, transformative. The characteristic property of fire is sight, mirroring the way in which our eyes are able to see into the darkness.

◊ **Water**, too, possesses sattvic qualities – when it's still, reflective, transparent and clarifying – yet it can also be impassable and immovable, which is tamas. The characteristic property of water is taste, via the tongue.

◊ **Earth** is pure tamas. It's the physical form, tangible and dense. The characteristic property of earth is smell, which we receive through the nose.

The Three Forces

There are also the three main forces at play within our external world – the sun, moon and wind. These all interplay with the Five Great Elements and the gunas and doshas (which we explore below) too.

◊ **The sun** – represented by the great element of fire – is the energy of transformation. Nothing can grow or survive without sunlight.

◊ **The moon** – whose silvery light quells and calms, and whose movements dictate the tides and cycles of our Earth – is both water and earth.

◊ **The wind** – with its relentless shifts and swirls – is an agent of motion and movement, and these are represented by both ether and air.

THE DOSHAS

The doshas are the three biological humours; they are comprised of differing ratios of the Five Great Elements:

◊ **Vata dosha** is characterized primarily by the wind (and to a lesser degree, ether): movement, airiness, lightness, flightiness.

◊ **Pitta dosha** is characterized mainly by fire (and to a much lesser degree, water): heat, passion, ambition, high energy.

◊ **Kapha dosha** is characterised by earth and water: cold, grounded, slow and steady – solid and reliable, with excellent stamina.

The sun relates to *Pitta* because Pitta is fire. On a searingly hot day, the sun causes Pitta to rise all around and within us – we may become red-faced, burn up, suffer heat rash or hives, or feel irascible, impatient, angry.

The moon, with its calming, stilling energy, relates to *Kapha*, which is both earth and water. When the moon is in the sky, we both slow and cool down, just as the tides swell and rise too – a beckoning towards the stillness and heaviness of sleep.

The wind is *Vata* at play – when the wind changes, things happen, driving movement and propelling us onwards; like rajas, postponing our stillness and rest.

The Doshas Through the Day

All is innate, subtlest harmony, with the rising and falling of energies to bring about a full 24-hour cycle between dawn and dusk.

Morning

Between 6 a.m. and 10 a.m., Kapha dosha is at its highest. The heavy, dull energy of Kapha isn't helpful when we seek to come into the day with vitality and lightness. Which is why Ayurveda recommends rising before sunrise (before 6 a.m., generally speaking), so that we may awaken before Kapha kicks in and seeks to pin us ever more immovably to our mattress.

From 10 a.m. into early afternoon (around 2 p.m.), our energy shifts to Pitta. This is a time of doing – more active, creative and motivated. Ayurveda suggests that much of the day's busy work be done between these hours (for those who have children at primary school, as we do, this will ring doubly true). We're supported at this time, with heightened clarity, intelligence and a sense of purpose.

Afternoon

After 2 p.m., the energy of the cosmos shifts yet again. When we might have felt positive and purposeful throughout the morning and early afternoon, the later part of the afternoon can leave us feeling unsure, a little lost, or overthinking things. Vata dosha is in full force now, and up to around 6 p.m., so the flighty energy of Vata causes us to lose our footing, second-guess, forget, question and doubt.

If you're in a position to take a walk at this time (a great way to generate new ideas), meditate on the task in hand, practise Yoga or simply sit, warm and comfortable, and do some deep-breathing exercises (try those shared in this book), it will help to counterbalance Vata's unsettling force.

Evening

The night, too, has its own rhythm, which mirrors that of the day. But now, instead, the best action becomes inaction. From 6 p.m. to shortly before 10 p.m. – a natural time of heightened Kapha – we're encouraged to embrace the languor and slowing of the senses. We're made to retreat, as the sun, too, prepares to set. So if you're in a position to slow down significantly during these hours, your body will most gratefully support your choice – and reward it with better sleep, which is the natural evolutionary aim of these slower, darker evening hours, after all.

This is the time to invite love, warmth and easy communion into the day – light and slow sattvic shared suppers with close friends and family, low voices, candlelight… you get the glowing picture.

Settling to sleep before 10 p.m. is the key note within this Vedic harmony too – we must make best use of Kapha's grounding, heavy, dulling energy if we want wonderfully sound and deep sleep.

Night-time

After 10 p.m., the energy picks up pace yet again, as the cosmos moves once more into Pitta time. This activating energy is often responsible for the 'second wind' we experience if we stay up past 10 p.m. (as almost all of us do at times), and carries on up to around 2 a.m., when we need to counterbalance the urge to 'do' with complete concession to rest. Ayurveda tells us to avoid any form of work at this time, to reduce stimulation to a minimum and to ensure we don't eat – to do so will stoke the fire of metabolism and send Pitta raging again (making it so much harder to sleep at all, once we do get to bed).

In the early hours, between 2 a.m. and up to 6 a.m., we move again into the variable, shifting energy of Vata – a less grounded, unsettled place. If you often wake up in the wee hours, you'll be familiar with Vata's flyaway, fretful energy. Sleep is the best antidote to excess Vata, but if it evades you, Vedic meditation and Yoga Nidra might help return you to a more restful, settled state.

We'll explore Vedic meditation later in the book; Yoga Nidra (also known as yogic sleep) involves lying in corpse pose – straight and comfortable on the floor – and following a guided meditation that takes the mind into a deepest state of relaxation. We are conscious, but in such a relaxed state that we're more deeply relaxed than in deepest sleep – a paradoxical conscious unconsciousness!

Morning

Then the cycle begins again, with earliest morning, before sunrise, rich with stillness and serenity: purest sattva, a time to be savoured.

Being aware of how these cosmic energies shift and blend, affecting all that we feel and are naturally inclined to do, is very liberating. Suddenly, we stop fighting the feelings, and learn their language instead.

GOD'S HOUR

Lying down to sleep at 10 p.m. and rising by 6 a.m. – mirroring the sun's rise – has brought us a new daily perspective. A peaceful home, stillest morning, time to breathe, listen to mantras, eliminate the previous day's waste, hydrate and, most importantly: sit and witness the sun rising within our world, and our selves, once more.

This is a deeply spiritual practice in Ayurveda, called *Brahma muhurta* ('the time of Brahma' – God's hour). We're gifted a daily opportunity to fill our cups, direct from the sun's life-giving light: to absorb this warmth, vitality and purest energy directly into our cells. Whenever we see it this way, it becomes that bit harder to choose the snooze button instead.

❧

Identify Your Dosha

In Ayurveda, we each have a unique constitution called our *prakriti*. It's the nature we're born with and it remains unchanged throughout our lives. Prakriti is our innate predisposition – how we're made and what makes us – and it reflects our tendencies and proclivities, according to the unique balance of the three doshas (Vata, Pitta, Kapha) within our selves.

Although our prakriti will never change, the way in which we're affected by daily energies and influences, and can be imbalanced by all that we do, say, think and eat, can temporarily affect our doshic make-up. That is our *vikriti* – our current state of imbalance. So, while you may be innately Pitta dosha – fiery, ambitious, hot-headed, passionate – there may be times in your life when you feel utterly demotivated, lethargic, heavy and passive, and this would be due to an imbalance of Kapha – although your prakriti is always Pitta, your vikriti may show a Kapha imbalance.

If you haven't already discovered your dosha, try the free test on our blog, This Conscious Life: www.thisconsciouslife.co/discover. The reason it's so helpful here is because knowing your prakriti and vikriti will help you to learn far more about those things that bring you back, and away from, your innate, natural harmony, and this also has rather a big impact on all aspects of your life.

To help you begin your journey towards discovering your prakriti, we've shared some simple descriptions of the doshas below. For most people, it's usually quickly apparent which 'type' they are, but many of us are a mixture of two (bi-doshic) and some people are an even mix of all three (tri-doshic).

Vata Dosha

If you're primarily Vata dosha, the elements that predominate within your body are space (or ether) and air. Not literally, but still, very evidently – in terms of how fast you speak, how many thoughts you quickly generate (and then promptly forget), and your flighty, airy, imaginative nature. You can be hard to pin down, often travelling; and you're airy in physique too, as Vata types are often thin, long-limbed and visibly bony.

You're not a deep sleeper – your mind is too busy swimming and flying – and your hunger wavers: sometimes ravenous, sometimes entirely lacking in appetite. Vata types tend to be artistic, creative and drawn to the performing and healing arts.

Restoring Balance to Vata

To balance your innate qualities of ether and air, choose rooting, grounding and slowing pursuits and energies – such as restorative Yoga and warm, lightly spiced and nourishing cooked foods that include spices such as cardamom, nutmeg, cinnamon and cumin, and root vegetables (avoid raw, cold and frozen). Consciously avoid that push to rush or race – two beautiful tonics for Vata types are barefoot walking and taking warm baths laced with grounding sesame oil and a few drops of ylang ylang, chamomile or frankincense essential oils.

Pitta Dosha

If you're primarily Pitta dosha, the elements of fire and, to a lesser degree, water, are your predominant forces. You literally feel hotter than most people and can be prone to heat-related imbalances such as heat rash, prickly heat and heartburn. Pitta types are driven, ambitious, charismatic and energetic. They tend to have a good, strong appetite and metabolism, sex drive and lust for life. Often athletic in build, with a sparkle to their paler-coloured eyes, Pitta types are most often our natural-born leaders.

Restoring Balance to Pitta

When Pitta is imbalanced, you can be hot-headed, irritable and impatient. If Pitta types don't quell their fire, they can quickly burn through their reserves (like an ever-accelerating car rapidly burning through petrol), and are left feeling quite suddenly depleted, shaky and feverish.

Pitta's natural prescription for restoring harmony includes cooling pursuits such as swimming and moonbathing (see page 45); herbal support from shatavari (a wonderful Pitta-balancing adaptogenic herb; see page 134); warm (not hot) baths laced with sunflower oil infused with rose and vetiver; reading gentle books and poetry; and listening to slow classical music.

Kapha Dosha

If you're primarily Kapha dosha, the elements of water and earth predominate in your body. You're naturally down-to-earth, grounded in your outlook and, often, a natural homebody. You're fond of your creature comforts, nurturing and stable in body and mind. Slow and steady gets the job done, and beautifully – Kaphas don't like to be rushed. Your body and hair tend towards lustre, sheen and softness, with generous curves and abundant embraces just two of your many gifts.

Restoring Balance to Kapha

Lethargy and heaviness can be felt when Kapha is imbalanced, though, so looking to energize and motivate yourself with pursuits that excite you and get the blood pumping are a wonderful choice. Add spice to your life, in all ways: from hiking with friends out in the fresh air, to disco dancing and fun-filled sexual frolics aplenty; seek out brilliant, enlivening acts to counterbalance your more steadfast nature, and look to shift stagnation with spicier foods, hot teas (ginger and turmeric are ideal) and naturally vitalizing essential oils such as cinnamon, eucalyptus and ginger.

SIMPLE SATTVIC SPI-RITUALS

With so many things to do, and so little time in which to do them, fundamental adjustments to our priorities have brought greater peace of mind, and living is now richer and easier in its flow. The following little rituals for the spirit – or 'spirituals' – draw on the deepest roots of Vedic knowledge, yet they are also some of the simplest things we've fallen in love with.

Reconnect with the Earth

In our 'every day', we increase our sattva by honouring and cultivating our connection with nature – by opening our minds and our intuitive urges to the shifts in the season, in the moon, sun and living world, and in our own rich inner world too. We take time outside in nature, every single day – even if it's just to sit on the doorstep, under the moonlit sky, during the evening of a particularly frantic day.

Most days, Paul spends at least a little time in the garden or at the allotment, listening to what's needed, responding, tending and harvesting. As often as we can, we camp out under canvas, get our feet back into the earth, wander through local woodland, swim in the sea and sit under the stars. Each and every time we do so, we're reminded of who we really are and what really matters – we come home.

Choose Silence Over White Noise

In the 21st-century Western world, sattva can be as simple as choosing to turn off the television and sit outside under a blanket and the light of the full moon – moonbathing, rather poetically, was once heartily recommended to those who were overly energized and frantic. Silver light – cooling and meditative – was seen as the cure-all for the fractious spirit.

It's so simple as to seem almost comical… yet it works. Often, at night, we get that urge for dullness – to sit numbly in front of a television rather than choosing restorative activities that really 'give back'. This feels like a natural antidote to a very challenging day – when so much is asked of us, we want to simply be left alone; the opposite of active: passive.

In winter, the urge to curl up under a blanket in front of the box is perhaps at its highest, and there's absolute joy to be had in favourite films and heartwarming dramas. But we'd suggest inviting sattva into life in other ways too. A fire lit in the hearth, candles dotted around the home, baths steaming and welcoming, accompanied by chai, cacao or fragrant tea – so that we may continue to warm our own cockles and light our own fires from within, even while weathering another stormy winter's night.

Nourish Your Needs

With our daily diet, we both listen in – responding to what our bodies, and those of our children, need and crave – and eat only those things that we really want. It's a great source of sadness for humanity that so often what we choose to eat isn't at all in tune with what we desire to eat, but rather a forceful diktat, borne of our fear around food. Fear that this food will make us fat or that food will make us unhealthy.

Much harmony comes from simply accepting every single one of your instincts, urges, cravings and desires – from telling your body (actively and out loud, if need be) that you are listening to it, that you love it and that you want to deeply, gently, kindly nourish it. When this harmony is restored, something quite miraculous, yet wholly natural, happens: your body softens as it sheds fear and guilt and anxiety around food, and you begin to make choices that come from deep within – intuitive, conscious choices based wholly upon what you now know your body needs.

That might be a hearty seasonal soup or the lightest, crunchiest, zesty salad, or an unctuous, cacao-rich, grounding mug of hot chocolate.

What we've also found, over and over again, is that the more we listen to our bodies and respond kindly, the more our bodies relax and are given permission to, once again, thrive. There's no battle to be fought between your wants and your perceived needs – Ayurveda sees nothing other than harmony in the non-existent space between mind, body, spirit – and by ignoring your own needs, you're creating disharmony, and eventually, the beginnings of dis-ease.

Meditate Your Way to Sattva

Even if just for 20 minutes a day, we both sit to meditate. When our routines are reliable (as they tend to be when our children are happy and healthy) we meditate early in the morning or later in the afternoon. We practice Vedic meditation, as taught to us by Will Williams (our wonderful UK-based teacher), but also use guided meditations and rounding techniques (an incredible ancient sequence of breath, asana, stillness and meditation), depending on the time we have, and what we crave, that day.

Meditation can truly be as simple as sitting in front of the rising sun for several minutes each morning, eyes closed, soaking up the warmth that imbues your skin – an offering to your body, now sun-warmed, softened, enlivened. Our children meditate too. There's no special room, place, moment, prop; they incorporate it into play and simply sit before bedtime and allow their sound to chime silently, to help the day's fray lift away and pave the way for more restful, easeful sleep.

Find Your Yoga

Yoga means many different things to many different people. For us, it's not the rigmarole of movement at a set time, in a set frame. It is, instead, simply an invitation to feel what we're feeling, and give back to our bodies and spirits what's needed. A simple round of sun salutations, which takes less than five minutes, never ceases to shift the night's stagnant energy: to free us up, heighten our awareness, soften our stiffness and invite yet more sattvic goodness – ease, harmony, contentment – into our lives.

Often, it's even simpler than that: an urge to drop to our knees and remain in Child's Pose, lungs expanding against thighs in what feels like a secure, love-locked embrace, forehead at one with the Earth. Back to nature, our nature – accepting that which we cannot change and choosing simply to be, instead.

The Magic of Massage

If we – or indeed our children – feel fractious, we take some time to massage one another. In the Ayurvedic tradition, children are massaged daily from one week of age up to the age of three; new mothers too, every day for 40 days after giving birth. Massage, or *abyhanga*, is seen as a truly sacred act in Ayurveda – a way of reminding ourselves of our various pieces and reuniting them all once more.

The physiological benefits of massage are well known in the West too – boosting circulation, improving the skin's quality, relieving stress… in Ayurveda, they go even deeper. Massage is an expression of love, and self-massage is an act of devotion. When we feel lost, sad, depleted, we can be brought back to a place of peace with the simple act of touch.

We enjoy making the simplest massage oils at home – adding a few drops of organic rose, sandalwood, frankincense or lavender essential oil to a base of cold-pressed sunflower or sesame oil, and then massaging this blend from the soles of the feet up to the shoulders. Rose oil, in particular, has long been prized for its ability to ease stress and dispel depression (and is widely supported by modern medical studies to this effect). It's been used in Ayurveda for centuries to help process emotions and ease the nervous system.

Eminé used rose-scented oils when pregnant and during labour, and continued with it during breastfeeding and beyond. So the sensual and scentual connection remains too – skin to skin – each time we massage it into and around the chest, with a focus on the heart; something our children adore too.

PRANAYAMA FOR HARMONY
– HUMMING BEE BREATHING

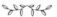

We've found that this, the *bhramari pranayama*, is a lovely evening practice, and it's wonderful as a preface to meditation. It promotes our inner awareness and brings harmony and relaxation to the mind. It's also restorative to the voice, so often in need of a little R&R. The humble humming of the black Indian bee. Let's begin:

1. Sit comfortably and upright, with awareness of your breathing and your head and neck erect.

2. Gently plug your ears with your index fingers and use your palms to cover your eyes; if your palms don't cover your eyes, simply close them.

3. Bring the tip of your tongue to touch the roof of your mouth, just behind your front teeth, with your jaw relaxed.

4. Breathe in deeply through the nostrils, ensuring that your abdomen inflates.

5. As you exhale slowly, make a low humming sound – beginning in your abdomen and vibrating in the back of your throat.

6. Continue to inhale and hum for as long as feels good. Be aware of any tension in the jaw and allow your body to relax.

MENSTRUAL HARMONY

Quite unique to Ayurveda is the insight and significance given to the menstrual cycle – indeed, if you've ever had a consultation with an Ayurvedic doctor you'll have answered many questions on it: from the quality and colour of the passing blood, to the sensations felt each time your cycle begins and ends.

This is because the menstrual cycle provides women with a uniquely valuable insight into the inner workings of their body. The spotlight is shone not just on the womb, but the other tissues of the body, too, including the plasma, the blood and all of the associated intricacies of the entire reproductive system – invaluable when looking to foster optimal holistic health.

The menstrual cycle also brings our attention, most acutely at times, to where we might need to make subtle changes, and begin to aid and rebalance our selves quite naturally too. In Ayurveda, period pain, cramping, bloating and excessive bleeding are seen as imbalances within the doshas that have manifested in the tissues of the body. To be clear – in Ayurveda, these symptoms point to disharmony within the body and are seen as being wholly avoidable and, in fact, unnatural.

In Ayurveda, menstruation is seen as a beautiful time of release and rebalance for all women; pain and depletion and extremely low mood should never be seen as our birthright – they are instead, symptoms of dis-harmony, readily righted by a return to the body's natural rhythms and deepest needs.

There are seven tissues, or structures, of the body (called *dhatus*). These are: the plasma, the blood, the muscle, the fat, the bone, the nerves and the reproductive tissue. They are always listed in this order, just as the Five Great Elements are always listed in their naturally evolving order: space (or ether) to air to fire to water to earth.

We can see, even with a cursory glance, that plasma might mirror space and reproductive tissue might mirror earth – again, it's micro mirroring macrocosm; the inner world as complex as the outer. How our inner balance and imbalances manifest will also affect the sort of period we have.

Each of the doshas plays its part in the menstrual cycle, at different times. Crucially, the pre-, post- and menstrual symptoms that may manifest in the body (from cramping and mood swings to increased appetite and sweating) will all directly relate to the balance (or imbalance) of the doshas in the body. The severity of symptoms is also greatly affected by the amount of *ama* (or toxins) that are held in the tissues, so one of the most important ways to restore sattva to the monthly cycle is to work gently to lighten the body's toxic load (we'll talk about this in more detail later).

Know Your Cycle

While everyone's cycle is different – and indeed, not all women bleed or experience their cycles in visible or traditional ways – the Ayurvedic advice for this most powerful of female cycles can help all of us who simply want to feel better acquainted with our inner landscapes and work towards restoring the body's innate rhythm and harmony.

In one of the earliest medical treatises, the *Charaka Samhita* (written in Sanskrit between 400 and 200BCE), there are lengthy passages on the reproductive cycle, which is described as lasting between 27 and 30 days. There are many Ayurvedic practitioners who also align the lunar cycle, 28.5 days, with the natural optimal length of the menstrual cycle (with ovulation historically occurring at the full moon and menstruation beginning at the new moon).

While there are many thousands of women who feel increasingly guided in their own menstrual cycles by the moon's shifting orbit – it can be extremely helpful in pre-empting mood and energy shifts, in particular – we'd like to encourage every single one of you reading this to do away with any and all comparisons or 'ideal' scenarios. Eminé often shifts from a red moon to a white moon cycle (red moon meaning that she menstruates when the moon is full; white when it's new).

These shifts can occur when life has been particularly imbalanced, challenging or frenetic. Eminé has also noticed that her cycle can swing between the full and new moons when there are big transitions in her life, or if she hasn't managed to spend much time outside in nature. Our cycles have been shown to naturally regulate far more efficiently when we expose ourselves to as much daylight as possible, simply because our hormones are affected by light and dark.

A variety of hormones, including melatonin, cortisol, thyroid-stimulating hormone (TSH) and prolactin (PRL), ebb and flow during the course of a single 24-hour day and are regulated by our circadian and sleep-wake cycles. So, simply spending more time outside during the day (with sunlight on the skin and light in the eyes) and then the converse – after sunset, minimizing our exposure to artificial light – will help to regulate our biorhythms and hormonal production, and is useful in bringing our cycles back to their natural norm (which, again, is different for us all).

Whenever you bleed (and if you've not bled regularly for some time), please know that every cycle is different and that we all begin in different places. By heeding the gentlest Ayurvedic advice later in this chapter, you can hope to move back to a place of inner harmony slowly and naturally, wherein your cycle will begin to self-regulate.

That is also why we've not proffered typical timings here for how long each part of the menstrual cycle ought to last. Some women bleed for two days, some seven; some ovulate early, others late; there's no right or wrong – you are the best reader of your body, and it functions optimally when there's as little outside interference as possible.

The Stages of Menstruation

In Ayurveda, the three main stages of the menstrual cycle possess their own unique characteristics, which relate to the shifts in hormones each time.

Rajahkala

During *rajahkala*, we menstruate. At this time we're in the Vata part of the menstrual cycle. This is because Vata is the energy that governs movement and flow, and Ayurveda encourages us to support the downward flow of this energy, so that we support our selves in the clearing of our menstrual blood from the body.

This is also why many Yoga teachers and Ayurveda practitioners discourage us from practising inversions while menstruating. There's a sense that we're impeding the body's natural rhythm and impetus – known as *apana vayu*: the subtype of Vata that governs downward flow and the gentle removal of urine and faeces too. In all that you do and feel at this time, remind yourself that it's healthy to let it out, let it go, let it be – this is a time of release and clearing, and your body feels that on every level.

Rutukala

After menstruation, Kapha is dominant. This part of the cycle, called *rutukala*, lasts from the end of the bleeding phase to the point at which we prepare to ovulate. The Kapha phase overlaps slightly with the Vata phase, as one part of the cycle segues into the next (much like the moon rising as the sun sets). During the Kapha phase, all of those typically Kapha energies come into play. The endometrium thickens (a sense of tending, nourishing and preparing the inner soil for what is to come), and we often feel fuller in our bodies at this time: softer, curvier, more supple – a beautiful realizing of our feminine energy.

Rutavateta kala

At the point of ovulation, we enter the Pitta phase of the cycle, or *rutavateta kala*. This is when the endometrium becomes fully engorged and filled with blood, ready to receive the ovum. We can feel warmer, more prone to sweating and increasingly hot-tempered at this time. Many women also feel a greater drive to do, create, socialize and achieve – the ambitious, motivating energy of Pitta supporting us at this time of the month.

If the ovum isn't fertilized, the cycle begins anew – with day one of menstruation, when the body once again clears and opens and we move, once more, into the Vata phase of our cycle.

Seen this way – the delicate flow from bleeding to receiving, from earthed and fleshy Kapha abundance to airy and cleansing Vata lightness – the body begins to feel more like intuitive symphonies of synergy and subtlety… and perhaps, if we begin to take a little more time to honour the magic behind the mechanics, we'll find our selves far more accepting of its highs and lows, ebbs and flows, too.

Menstruation and the Doshas

Sattva, being the very essence of harmony and serenity, can feel laughably removed from many of our physical and emotional experiences of the menstrual cycle – the intricacies and intimacies of which are far too complex and individual to be addressed amply here. Yet, there is much comfort to be taken in knowing that a natural, healthy menstrual cycle should never be a source of pain or sadness.

Ayurveda describes a healthy period as the passing of bright red blood without clots, which rinses easily away from cloth or clothing (if your bleed produces stubborn stains, it's a sign that the blood contains toxins, or ama, and it's an important sign to heed). The smell, too, should be natural and bodily but never unpleasant or foul.

While every cycle plays out in the same way, from Vata-Kapha-Pitta states as we move from menstruation to post-ovulation, it's yet more individualized than that too. As we mentioned earlier, the three doshas can manifest in the tissues of the body and cause dosha-specific imbalances that affect the menstrual cycle and how it *feels*. We explore each dosha and how it manifests during your menstrual cycle – and, hearteningly, what you can do to bring natural balance and sattvic calm into your month.

Vata Menstruation

Vata types are the most likely to experience scant, absent and painful periods. This is due to the effect of Vata on the blood vessels – constricting, cooling, tightening. When we bleed, our bodies seek release, so we want Vata's opposite: to dilate, open up and let go. So when Vata is heightened, we can see how the imbalance impedes the body's natural urge. Vata also naturally resides within the pelvic space, and if the imbalance isn't addressed it's common for Vata types to experience depletion of the tissues, which can present as outer emaciation.

For Vata types who lose weight very easily, particularly when anxious and frantic, periods can stop for a while too: the tissues of the body being no longer nourished, moist and supple enough to support flow. Blood, when it does come, is often darker in colour – a sign that older blood from a previous cycle has mixed with fresher blood, and that, once again, the flow from the uterus is stymied in some way.

Restoring Harmonious Flow to Vata

Ayurveda is a beautiful dance of harmonizing opposites. To counter-balance the dry, cool, sparse qualities of Vata, we want to overnourish, lubricate, feed, ground, warm and soften, on every level. Return to those comfort foods of childhood – soft, mushy, soothing, warming, fragrant. Well-cooked soups, stews, curries (a yielding marigold-yellow tarka dal is a failsafe), made with plenty of butter, coconut, sesame oil or best of all, ghee, will feed those tissues up from within.

Switch from coffee (Vata needs rooting, not enervating) to soothing, warming teas – cardamom, cinnamon and, best of all, sweet, gently spiced milks: golden turmeric milk and chai are gifts to the Vata body. There are harmonizing adaptogenic herbs and spices too, more widely available today in the West – shatavari (see page 134), bala and gokshura are wonderful Vata-balancers.

Traditionally, these herbs are added to ghee to form a medicated butter, which can then be stirred through milk (as with turmeric in golden milk) and drunk. A beautiful, enriching and nourishing way to feed up those Vata-weakened tissues, but also understanding of the fact that most herbs and spices, and vitamins and minerals too, are lipid-soluble, so we increase the amount of goodness that the body can absorb when we choose to eat or drink such things with a little fat.

To ease pain, warm and loosen the muscles and tissues as much as you can. Japanese haramaki wraps are practical and comfortable – a soft band of material that keeps the core warm on the coldest days. Ayurveda's equivalent is a castor oil pack. Although it's not recommended that you use a pack while menstruating, they are ideal in the days that lead up to menstruation. The qualities of castor oil are heating and unctuous – a natural antidote to Vata.

Soak a long length of fabric that you've chosen for the purpose and won't need to use for anything else (muslin, cotton, wool) in warm castor oil, wring out and then wrap around the pelvis. You can choose to place a hot-water bottle on top to increase the heat pack sensation, or leave the warming castor oil to do that for itself. Castor oil washes out easily enough, but if lying down, it's worth putting a towel underneath you, and also wearing old clothes on top while you take this time to rest. Indeed, rest also plays a crucial role in harmonizing the Vata cycle.

Naturally get-up-and-go light sleepers and creative beings, overthinking Vata types need to be given permission to slow, stop, curl up, hibernate and sleep. Sleep elevates our rooted, earthy, heavy Kapha dosha – which is, yet again, the natural counterbalancing anchor to Vata's feather-lightness, moved by every wind that blows.

Pitta Menstruation

With the heat and flow and force of Pitta (characterized by the fire and water elements), Pitta cycles are often heavy, and they can begin quickly, with bleeding coming on all of a sudden. Along with the heat comes the obvious rise in temperature (many Pitta types feel extremely hot and bothered in the lead-up to and early days of their period), tenderness and swelling – particularly in the breasts. With the rush of flow and increased heat in the tissues, Pitta types are also more likely to have looser bowel movements, even diarrhoea, during their period; many, too, can feel nauseous.

Restoring Harmonious Flow to Pitta

One of the most important ways for Pitta types to balance their own inner fire during their heavy cycles is to lighten up in all other ways. That means a removal from competitive, aggressive, overly challenging activities and behaviours – and any activity that really gets the blood up (they have more than enough blood already!) In the same vein, spicy, overly rich, oily and salty foods will all continue to stoke the inner fire, when it needs the opposite: quelling and cooling.

Coconut oil and milk, mint, nettle, lavender, chamomile and coriander are all cooling additions and can be used freely in whatever combinations are desired. Because of the rush and force of bleeding with Pitta types, there can be a real feeling of sudden depletion. If the blood contains toxins (ama) the flow can be painful and unpleasant too.

In Ayurveda, organic aloe vera juice is recommended as a natural blood cleanser and excellent cooling tonic – sip a small glass twice a day, on an empty stomach. Other herbs that support harmony of the Pitta cycle include brahmi (also known as gotu kola) and shatavari (see page 134), both of which quell Pitta's excessive fire, bringing stability and sattvic balance back to the reproductive tissues.

Kapha Menstruation

With the elements of earth and water, Kapha is the heaviest and most lethargic of the doshas. This slow flow and stagnating quality can make it difficult for things to move through the body in a healthy way, and Kapha types are most likely to retain fluid, bloat, swell and suffer distention of the bowel and abdomen. Periods can last longer for them, and blood is often thicker, stickier and heavier. A desire to sleep more also pervades, but, sadly for Kapha types, this will only exacerbate lethargy.

Restoring Harmonious Flow to Kapha

Working once again with the natural law of opposites, we seek out lightness and fluidity. If the body is overly damp and cold inside – which brings about those sluggish feelings, and the slow flow of fluid too – it needs to be warmed up, excited, energized.

Agni, the fire that transforms and enlivens us (and also drives metabolism), needs dedicated stoking now. Kapha types should add more spice to their daily food – black pepper, cinnamon, ginger (fresh ginger tea is a wonderful tonic all month long for them), and avoid sweet, stodgy, heavy foods (processed, fried and overly oily foods in particular, which slow the bodily processes even more); meat, yoghurt and cheese are highly Kapha-elevating too.

Kapha types should choose light broths, zingy soups, spiced pulse and bean curries and stews, and Ayurvedic teas of tulsi (also known as holy basil), cardamom, turmeric and cinnamon. They can bring heat into the body from the outside too, with warming castor oil wraps (as described earlier, for Vata types, and as before, these should be used prior to, but not during, menstruation) and hot baths with four to five drops of either ginger, cedar, cinnamon or clove essential oils.

It's helpful for Kapha types to move more in the run-up to menstruation too. Try brisk strolls, hiking, running – the aim is to increase the rate of flow and shift stagnation: to wake up the body. Stimulate the natural excretory process with daily dry body brushing, or natural, exfoliating scrubs. Slightly more dynamic forms of Yoga (such as *kundalini*, which awakes the fire in the belly – wonderful for Kapha – or *vinyasa*, which brings heat into the tissues) and deep, cleansing breathing (pranayama) will support Kapha well at this time too.

MOTHER NATURE'S CYCLES

Ayurveda has brought Eminé a huge amount of insight into her own natural reproductive cycle, and since paying more attention to the balance within her body, month by month, she's not only managed to alleviate symptoms of PMS, but has also come to respect her body in a way that she'd not necessarily thought a great deal about in her youth.

Within nature, there are many, many natural cycles – birth to death, full to new moon, receding to advancing tides, ovulation to menstruation – and each one happens according to its very own rhythm. These gentle harmonies can be easily upset – women's cycles are highly sensitive and shocks to our system can quickly knock them off-course.

We don't expect flowers to stay in bloom year-round, yet with the female body, which experiences continual, completely natural changes in hormone levels and significant changes throughout the course of the year (we're plunged into our own inner winter when we come to bleed each month), we somehow expect our selves to remain constant – regardless of the myriad changes that happen in and all around us.

If we choose to regulate or even eternalize our menstrual cycle – for example, by taking the contraceptive pill for a long stretch of time without a break – we're also choosing force over flow, and chemically inducing the body to do something that it would never naturally do.

While it may seem benign enough to skip a period for fear that it may 'spoil' a special day, there are many women who see all periods as things to be ignored, loathed or wholly avoided, if at all possible. An inconvenient truth. To do so, however, is to deny a vital part of what makes you a biological miracle – a woman. We recommend some wonderful reading material on the female body and menstrual cycle in the Sattvic Resources section, and we do hope you'll dip in (or better yet, imbibe, with gusto).

AYURVEDA DURING MENOPAUSE

Menopause (*Rajonivritti*) is medically defined as a full year with the absence of a period. In the run-up to menopause, it's common for women to experience symptoms caused by decreasing levels of the hormone oestrogen – from hair thinning and breast tenderness, to heightened irritability and night sweats – which can last from anywhere between one and 10 years.

These 'perimenopausal' symptoms, which we typically associate with 'menopause', are, then, not typically menopausal at all: they are signposts along the path of natural transition and, according to Ayurveda, if one begins to prepare the body for menopause long before it naturally occurs, the experience should be a far gentler and more positive one.

Ayurveda heralds menopause as a time of release, liberation and deepest transformation – into a period of life built upon a foundation of wisdom and experience. During menopause, we transition from a Pitta to a Vata phase of life. If Pitta or Vata dosha are imbalanced and particularly high, symptoms will also be heightened. In the run-up to menopause, then, it's important to focus on balancing Pitta (those typical hot flushes of perimenopause can be quelled with a Pitta-pacifying diet and lifestyle – more below), and as we move closer to menopause, when Vata rises, shifting our lifestyles so that they nourish, root, ground and support our bodies, is recommended.

Managing Pitta During Perimenopause

As is true of all of Ayurveda, seeking to treat symptoms is never as effective as achieving balance at a foundational level – long before the symptoms appear. In order to keep the body balanced and symptom-free during perimenopause, Ayurveda advises women who seek a peaceful and positive menopausal experience to adopt regular lifestyle protocols and regimens in their late 20s to early 30s.

This isn't overly cautious, but simplest good sense. A woman can observe both a healthy daily regimen (*dinacharya*) and a seasonal regimen (*ritucharya*): adapting her lifestyle to naturally counterbalance the shifts in the seasons, and keeping her body clear, balanced and healthy with *Pancha Karma* (if, for example, a dosha has been aggravated and needs thorough rebalancing; see section on Pancha Karma, page 101). The upshot is a woman who is in optimal health: vital, healthy, balanced and strong. And, when her time comes, such a woman would be far less likely to experience negative symptoms during menopause, simply because her body is low in ama, and her doshas are harmonized.

To balance Pitta, all of the earlier advice in this chapter applies. Ayurveda also specifies a type of Pitta that resides in the liver – *Ranjaka Pitta*. If liver function is compromised due to an ongoing excessive level of Pitta within the liver, then the direct and crucial role this organ plays in metabolizing and ridding the body of excess hormones will be far less effective. An optimally functioning liver is a real cornerstone of optimal menopausal health, and to restore balance to this vital excretory organ, it's important to consider the following things:

Avoid foods that raise Pitta – e.g. spicy, fried, salty, very sour foods, alcohol and caffeine. All are greatly Pitta-elevating.

Invite calmer, slower and more soothing activities into your life. A great deal of research has been done into the positive effects of both Yoga and meditation on perimenopausal symptoms and menopause. Rush less, juggle less, do less – build in daily swathes of stillness, silence, fresh air and nature. Dampen your excessive fire with cooling moonlight, time beside water, gentle classical music, soothing bedtime reading and quality sleep.

Managing Vata During Menopause

In her book *The Ageless Woman*, Nancy Lonsdorf says: "In tribal and rural India, women living simple, low-stress lives rarely have menopausal problems. Physical exertion and a diet of fresh foods (especially wild yam), grains such as quinoa and amaranth, and spices with estrogenic effects all have a modulating or balancing effect on hormone levels."[1]

In the West, however, such a life is not the norm. Stress is rife – and chronically high cortisol levels are almost always indicated in women who struggle most during menopause. Given that heightened Vata is typical of this menopausal period, it is, again, important to consider all the ways in which we can balance this dosha. To nourish and rebuild the tissues (dhatus) and *Ojas*, the sweet flavour is best. Food should be warming, soupy, substantial and high in good natural fats – to counteract the Vata-caused dryness that we see so often when this dosha predominates. Cooked grains, cereals and pseudo-cereals (amaranth and quinoa being wonderful), sweet root vegetables, and warming oils such as sesame and olive, feed up the body and root it in goodness.

Lifestyle factors and a daily regimen are equally important. Vata benefits most of all the doshas from sitting in stillness to eat – slowly,

---

1   Lonsdorf MD, Nancy, *The Ageless Woman*; MCD Century Publications, 2004

to savour, chew and absorb. Characteristically 'busy' in mind and body, by introducing a regular eating routine, rooted in one place, with slow-cooked meals and thought given to how we nourish our selves, we automatically counterbalance Vata's urge to be always 'on the go'.

Another enriching lifestyle practice for women in menopause is massage therapy (see page 48). The act of slowing for long enough to massage warm oil into the entirety of the body is not only a sweetest salve for our skin, tissues and senses, but a deeply balancing spi-ritual too. It lowers Vata simply by virtue of being Vata's opposite: slow, languid, warm and tactile.

A 2010 study[2] on the use of rejuvenative Ayurvedic herbs (*rasayana* herbs) also showed that the Ayurvedic herbal medicine Saraswatarishta promoted measurable improvements in the psychological wellbeing of menopausal women who had previously been experiencing symptoms of anxiety, depression and 'emptiness'. Saraswatarishta is a liquid medicine that supports immunity, physical strength, good memory, longevity and a healthy libido. It contains several powerful adaptogenic Ayurvedic herbs, including brahmi, shatavari, haritaki (from the seeds of the terminalia chebula tree) and vidari (a relative of wild yam).

---

2   Santwani, K., et al, 2010. 'An assessment of *Manasika Bhavas* in menopausal syndrome and its management'. www.ncbi.nlm.nih.gov/pmc/articles/PMC3221064

Herbs for Menopause

Highly recommended for women in menopause is the uterine tonic shatavari, phyto-oestrogen-rich wild yam, liquorice, the stress-relieving adaptogen ashwagandha, naturally liver- and gut-cleansing triphala, brahmi, gotu kola and amla (commonly known as Indian gooseberry). As with all Ayurvedic herbs and tonics, we highly recommend seeking out a professional practitioner, for which the Ayurvedic Practitioner's Association (the APA) are an excellent resource.

Herbs following a Hysterectomy

For those women who have had a hysterectomy, their uterus – the seat of their biological fire, and also their metabolic fire, or agni – has been removed, and for many women, this equates to an extremely natural, deeply rooted feeling of real loss: emotional, psychological and physical. After a hysterectomy many women might also begin to feel less motivated, less positive and begin to lack their customary lust for life. Ayurveda can be very helpful in supporting women to rebuild their vitality (Ojas) – and shatavari is highly prized here because it restores sattva, counteracts stress and promotes natural hormonal balance. Indeed, even after a hysterectomy, the body continues to produce a little oestrogen, so taking a natural adaptogenic herb such as shatavari, which supports oestrogen production, is a very positive step for all women.

THE HARMONIOUS HOME

There's an entire branch of Vedic science dedicated to architecture, the art of the harmonious environment and the placement of all things within it: Vastu Shastra. While the science is complex, and we're limited here by space, it's a lovely thing to consider when looking to cleanse and clear the energy of the home, and create a place where we don't only live, but truly thrive.

Simple shapes were attributed to the energies that might preside in a home. The inert heaviness of tamas was represented by the unbreakable circle, which mirrored the solidity of 'earth'; the active, propelling force of rajas was represented by the triangle; and sattva, with its harmonious qualities, was the stable and balanced square – the ideal shape for our homes (with the rectangle seen as a more than suitable alternative).

Given that very few of us will have the funds to commission a 'grand design' from scratch, we'll work here with the obvious modern-day constraints of the homes we'll likely purchase (most of which, happily, tend to come in rectangular configurations). Having said this, many of us have already felt the 'energy' of a space – perhaps when we crossed the threshold of the home we now inhabit – and felt welcomed, buoyed, optimistic, calm, or the opposite: repelled, uncomfortable and keen to leave as quickly as we could. It's this feeling that underlies much of what we share here – a sense of inviting the good energy in and warding off the unwanted.

In Vastu Shastra, basic quadrants of the home are assigned different purposes; this makes sense because we wouldn't want to entertain guests or work intensively in the same space in which we'd then hope to get a peaceful, uninterrupted night's sleep.

When you fall asleep with your head pointing north, it's said that you're positioned in opposition to the Earth's natural magnetic fields, which flow from north to south; like repelling like. Having your head face any other direction is considered preferable (facing east is said to be best for improving memory and concentration; while south and west were historically said to bring good health and wealth). We've also enjoyed sleeping with our heads facing east, as we then benefit from the natural position of the rising sun – a beckoning from Mother Nature to rise early, more easily and with increased energy.

Honouring the Elements and Energies

Even if modern life precludes the creation of Vastu Shastra-optimized conditions, we still have conscious choice on our side, and likewise, with the way in which we honour the Five Great Elements (ether/space, air, fire, water and earth) within our home: another cornerstone of Vastu Shastra. Traditionally, the god of fire, Agni, was said to be positioned in the southwest corner of the home, so one would place the hearth, fire, or stove there; likewise, Varuna, the god of water, was said to be positioned in the westerly corner, where one would install the bathing room.

For us, again, there's a conscious nod towards the keeping of energies and elements in their rightful place – our bathroom, a place of real sanctuary but also purifying ritual, is kept very separate in its functions from the rest of our lives. According to Vastu, toilets were always kept entirely separate from living accommodation (one would bathe in a room that didn't contain a toilet). Of course, this was at a time when human waste didn't politely pass into sanitized waterways, so it was pragmatic to put some room between your self and your waste.

If you've ever taken your phone into the bathroom with you – perhaps to pass the time – you're certainly mixing and muddling opposing energies. The only business that ought to happen in the bathroom is your body's business; it's a place to answer nature's call (and nature's call alone). It's also worth mentioning that those 'hole-in-the-ground' toilets prevalent in India and elsewhere, which some might consider 'basic' or unpleasant, encourage an optimal squatting position for effective elimination. The 'thrones' we chair-centric Westerners use may be easier, but they place more strain on our back passage. Keeping a low stool by the toilet on which to place your feet makes for more effective positioning.

DESIGN FOR YOUR DOSHA

In accordance with Vastu Shastra, the rooms in a home are always clean, clear of clutter, well ventilated and full of natural light – balanced with cooler rooms to provide shelter from the sun. The purpose of the home is indistinguishable from the *feeling* of the space.

Kapha Dosha

Earthier and beautifully grounded Kapha types tend to be real homebodies – more likely to nest, sleep in and choose home over a night out. Yet, if left unchecked, this natural urge can move into lethargy and that comforting blanket of home can move towards a tendency for reclusiveness. Creating a home that enlivens your senses and warms your heart – bringing glow to your naturally colder Kapha body – will help immeasurably.

Avoid neutral or monochromatic palettes: they don't excite your senses. Look, instead, for sunny shades – red, amber, terracotta, yellow or gold – and use them as generously as you like, to bring a heartening warmth into your home.

While Kapha types tend to be good, deep sleepers, look to keep your bedroom as airy and clutter-free as possible (as clutter increases tamas and heaviness). Try to bring a feeling of 'spice' to the bedroom too, with tactile fabrics, furnishings, candles and warm metallic accents. Indeed, give free rein to your imagination and conjure as many variations of 'spice' as you care to: more sex is a wonderful balancer for the languor that can take hold of slow and steady Kapha types.

Pitta Dosha

For Pitta types, who are easily overexcited and prone to burning the candle at both ends (driven, as they are, to succeed), it's crucial to create a haven where work and home lives are clearly delineated. Be strict with your technology – and keep your phones and devices well away from the areas in which you rest and sleep. Clear clutter and things that tempt you to return to work once you ought to be done for the day, and surround yourself with sattvic living houseplants (see Cleansing with Air, page 89) and lots of balancing natural light.

If you're a fiery Pitta type, it also makes sense to invite cooling colours and materials into the home – from silvery blues, pale greens and moon-infused hues, to paler wood, cotton, bamboo or linen sheets, and touches of silk to calm the heat of your body.

Vata Dosha

For Vata types, where the energy is very much up and away with the air and ether, the home is of crucial importance – a place to root, nest, slow and rest, as often as you can. Pay particular attention to your bedroom: Vata types often give greater priority to their working or socializing rooms, but this is indicative of how little they can value their sleep. Make it as welcoming as you can, with thick, tactile fabrics (wool knits, cashmere, alpaca) and the warmest bedclothes (don't be tempted to sleep under thin sheets in an exposing slip – it may be the stuff of Hollywood movies, but it makes for a particularly shivery and flighty Vata).

The Living Space

In the living space, we want to heighten the soothing energy of sattva as much as we can. Care is taken to avoid introducing anything into the environment that's negative or violent in connotation – this could be anything from the watching of aggressive films to the hanging of artwork that depicts tumultuous scenes, or invokes some form of violence (paintings of storms or natural disasters; portraits of predatory animals; taxidermy). Sattva in the mind is only accessed from a place of stillness and gentleness.

In the West, our living rooms are often centred entirely around our television sets, and we often regard watching TV as a form of relaxation: a way to 'switch off' because we're physically still and passive. As we said earlier, in truth, television watching is the opposite of switching off. While it's passive in the sense that we're not contributing to the outcome in front of us, we're still very much being stimulated by those flashing images that pass before our eyes.

This isn't coming from a place of sanctimony. It's undeniably commonplace in our modern world, with its appetite for thrillers, crime and violence, to spend an evening watching a programme that unsettles and disturbs us – from the pounding adrenalized heart as we sit in fear of something terrible happening, to the visceral feeling of violation as we watch something that truly upsets us.

While we may be watching fiction (or indeed not – the daily news can be the most unsettling viewing of all), we must also be aware of the effects that our chosen material is having on our minds and spirits. The same is true of the books and newspapers we choose to read; at the end of a busy or challenging day, are we too often seeking out another state of fear or panic – 'addicted' to the adrenaline rush of a thrilling, frightening story when we should, ideally, be experiencing rest and replenishment?

Even if we choose to sit and enjoy an hour of the BBC's *Gardeners' World* – with its deeply soothing and uplifting images of nature – this is still removed from the Vedic ways within which we'd truly have transcended the ever-thinking and processing mind and touched upon that still and pure state of sattva. For example, via the practice of Vedic meditation, mantra or Yoga Nidra, where the mind is brought to a point of stillness – away from the rambles and worries, catastrophizing and panic, overthinking and forecasting. Into the absoluteness of the here and now: nothing before, nothing beyond. Just peace.

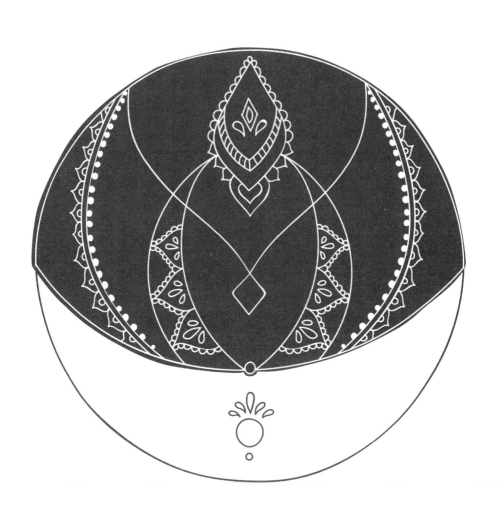

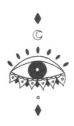

CHAPTER 3

PURITY

'Because we cannot scrub our inner body we need
to learn a few skills to help cleanse our tissues,
organs, and mind. This is the art of Ayurveda.'

SEBASTIAN POLE

NATURE PURIFIES US – fresh, clean air, oxygenating plants, naturally antibacterial oils. And, because we, too, are 'nature', we possess all that we need to cleanse our selves effectively and gently too: from our powerhouse vital organs and homeostatic mechanisms, to our wisest natural instincts, where we are well guided by intuition and sensorial curiosity.

In this chapter, we explore the natural sattvic ways in which our bodies can be supported, cleansed and healed, and our homes and spaces cleared and energized – under Mother Nature's watchful and supportive eye. While 'clean' and non-toxic living isn't our focus here (and talk of 'chemicals' is also misleading as oxygen, nitrogen, hydrogen and carbon are all chemical elements, and all wholly natural too), we've learned a lot about what it means to live in a conscious, ethical and kind way.

SATTVA AT HOME

Sattvic living is about edging ever closer to what feels intuitively good and right. For us, sattva at home is a subtle thing that boils down to the natural resonance of natural materials – it just *feels* better.

At home, we're trying, ever more consciously, to invite in only those things with which we feel a natural affinity. This mirrors the choice we long ago made for our bodies too – never to consume plastic-wrapped, ready-made, microwavable fast food or sugar-laden carbonated drinks, and to nourish our selves with fresh, vital, seasonal choices, every day. Purity for us really means simplicity – choices uncomplicated by 'unnecessaries'.

When we bake bread, we need only three ingredients for a beautiful loaf, so why, when we buy it, does it contain 20? When we moisturize our bodies with oil – perhaps the cold-pressed sunflower oil that we infuse with our homegrown calendula flowers, which stays fresh and nourishing for upwards of a year in its vivid blue glass bottle – why, when we buy moisturizer, does it require half a dozen different preservatives and a base of inert petrochemicals?

By paring back and cleansing away the things we no longer need – and there's real power in separating what we *really do* need from what we've been led to *believe* we need – we begin, quite naturally, to cleanse not just the home we live in, but the energies that pervade it too.

We give thought to each and every thing we bring into our home: from the reclaimed wooden bench that has become the heart of the busy living area (school bags lined up; shoes slipped on; post sorted through), to the old oak larder that we found on eBay for a song and now fill with our flour, pasta, pulses, cereals and other dried goods.

Plastic water bottles, that most environmentally inconvenient of conveniences, have been swapped out for life-lasting stainless steel and glass, while food is wrapped in paper, cloth or eco wrap. We long ago rid our home of bleach and cleaning chemicals (as an asthmatic child, Eminé can still remember the coughing fits she'd have at school, where the smell of bleach pervaded every classroom and corridor), and use a mixture of shop-bought natural cleaners, washable cloths and homemade concoctions (varying combinations of bicarbonate of soda, Castile soap, essential oils and vinegar will do almost every household job).

We burn natural incense and candles, travel light and carry spare cotton totes in all of our various bags (and in the boot of our family car). We grow a lot of our own veg, herbs, helpful flowers and fruit too – outside in our little garden and on our allotment plot – and each time we gather these natural gifts into our hands, that connection with the Earth resonates through us too. When there's a deficit, we've a few favourite foraging spots, local farms and shops we like to visit.

With a lot of good local stuff on our doorstep we're lucky, and for the purposes of economy we've always made good use of the local supermarket too, where it's easier than ever to carry over our conscious choices – we were so happy to find inexpensive jaggery (our unrefined sweetener of choice) and value packs of basmati rice, mung dal and dried pulses in the 'world food' section. Spices contribute so often to our little doshic adjustments, and make it much easier to improvise a delicious, simple, sattvic meal at the drop of a hat, so it's well worth stocking up on as many as you can afford, and enjoy.

CLEANSE YOUR SPACE

Tamas, as previously discussed, is the weight of the solid and physical – possessions and obligations among them. It weighs on us literally and figuratively – heavy bags, overstuffed; possessions with their life-long payment plans. Sattva, then, is the impetus that takes us away from our earthly possessions and their burdening qualities, towards a space where things are light, clear, pure.

If Mother Nature blesses us with those highest qualities of sattva each time the sun rises, we can invite that energy into our homes far more effectively if our windows are clean, our sills clear and our curtains flung open to their widest point. The sattvic home is a welcoming space filled with ease, light and fresh air, rather than trinkets, trophies, teetering piles and unwanted tokens.

Begin at the beginning. Assess what you no longer need – what burdens your senses, what brings a feeling of heaviness (whether in the form of financial obligation or a sense of spiritual suppression) into your home – and make a conscious choice. Could you donate it to someone who can make much better use of it? Can you take it to a recycling centre or charity shop? If it's natural, non-toxic and burnable (e.g. piles of old non-coated paper and dismantled cardboard boxes), add it to the fire – it's free fuel for the wood burner, or you can use it as the bones of an outdoor *puja*, should you wish to create a space-clearing ritual at home (more on this coming up).

If you sense that your home has an unwelcome 'feeling' about it – as though there's some sort of energy trapped or stagnating that you cannot quite put your finger on – it's important to address this. Recently, many people have re-embraced ancient cultural cleansing methods such as smudging – burning sacred herbs and resins including palo santo (wood from the holy palo santo tree, which is native to North America) and sage (white or blue, and grown specifically for purpose) – to clear, not just the physical air (as many of these plants are naturally antibacterial), but the spiritual space too.

However, we feel it's just as important to know where these rituals originated, for which purpose and how best to invite them into your own home.

Aromatherapy

Aromatherapy has become hugely popular in the West, and awareness of just how many benefits can be gained from nature's cornucopia, and how versatile essential oils are in their usage, from topical to internal, has grown substantially in the 21st century.

Ayurveda has always utilized natural aroma, and in a way that understood the multifarious effects of these potent fragrant substances – on not only the body, but the mind and spirit too. In terms of the physical purification of space, there are many herbs that can effectively cleanse the home, all of which will have a very happy knock-on effect on the body, mind and spirit; basil essential oil, for instance, will not only imbue the air with awakening scent, but will purify it too, bring clarity to the mind, and sharpen the senses (office managers and head teachers, take note).

Indeed there are many essential oils that can help to support our immune system, as they are extremely useful in the treating of infections, and many have also proven to be effective in killing pathogens. In many instances, the oil itself will let us know its uses – think of the pungent herb eucalyptus, with its menthol-like ability to open up the nasal passages. Simply inhaling it seems to expand our lungs, clear the mind and dispel sluggishness – a breath of fresh air. This tangible effect on us is mirrored by the qualities that Ayurveda attributes to it: as good for stagnation, toxicity, phlegm and congestion. Dr David Frawley also describes it as cleansing the psychic air. Pay attention – your intuition will often guide you well here.

FIVE PURIFYING AROMAS

Thyme Oil

With its natural antiseptic and antiparasitic properties, this is a very useful oil to have at home. Ayurveda merits thyme's usefulness at warding off airborne viruses and protecting the lungs – it's a good one to call upon during cough, cold and flu season.

Patchouli Oil

This is good for dispelling extreme lethargy and sluggishness – when Kapha types are in need of rebalancing, perhaps; it's therefore also good at lifting deep, dark, low moods and helpful for depression. As it's pungent, patchouli oil is also useful in shifting cold, damp conditions within the body – mucous and phlegm – and is helpful for the digestive system, stimulating appetite and agni.

Myrrh

A tree resin rather than a plant oil, myrrh is highly prized in Ayurveda. Often used in cleansing rituals, it can be placed on charcoal and burned (as can frankincense resin and pine resin). It possesses many different actions, being classed as pungent, bitter and astringent, with slight sweetness too. Its purifying actions are manifold: its antifungal and antimicrobial properties make it a potent blood cleanser in Ayurveda, and modern research has explored its promising anti-tumour potential too.[3] It can also be used diluted as a mouthwash, for oral health. Gargling with it has been shown to help with gingivitis and expedite the healing of mouth sores and ulcers.

Cedar Oil

Commonly called cedarwood in the West, this oil is cleansing and antiseptic. It's a wonderful oil to add to diffusers and oil burners at home, and is useful in clearing the lungs and opening up a wider sense of 'space' if energy feels stagnant; it's also an efficacious (and pleasingly scented) oil to add to household disinfectant cleaning sprays.

Basil

As previously mentioned, basil is very highly valued in Ayurveda for its ability to cleanse the air, the airways, the lungs, and the mind and spirit too. It's thought to create space within the home – it's ideal as a devotional tool, and to burn when there is a lingering sense of tension or negativity.

---

3   al-Harbi M.M. et al, 1994. 'Anticarcinogenic effect of Commiphora molmol on solid tumors induced by Ehrlich carcinoma cells in mice'. www.ncbi.nlm.nih.gov/pubmed/7956458

Holy basil, or tulsi, is different to the commonly found basil grown in the West, but the latter is still in possession of wonderful purifying properties. The Ayurvedic sages recommended keeping a holy basil plant within the home – ideally in a space where we meditate, or require clarity of mind, energy and purpose.

Purifying with Fire and Smoke

Agni is the Vedic god of fire and also the literal word for fire; agni is also the word we use for our own internal metabolic heat and digestive fire. What the word also embodies is the very idea and principle of transformation – so, fire is seen as the truly holy and profound element it really is.

In Vedic traditions, there are many forms of fire ritual – all rooted in the belief that fire brings about transformation. This impetus towards higher consciousness and purity of spirit is beautifully sattvic – the phoenix rising from the ashes, enlightened, unburdened, reborn.

The Ritual of Homa

Vedic fire ceremonies have many names and specificities. *Homa* is the Sanskrit word for a ritual that involves fire; the Hindu word is *yajna* or *yagna*. Rather than a sacrificial ritual, homa is a votive offering to the god of fire, Agni – traditionally, foods such as ghee, grains, herbs and seeds would have been placed into the fire – to honour and give thanks for life's goodness and blessings, but also in the hope of being kept in the god's good graces.

The ritual of homa highlights the fire's ability to take earthy offerings and make them divine – only when the votives had been transformed by the fire were they then conveyed up to the heavens, via the reams of rising smoke, as fit for the gods.[4] Today, in the comfort of our homes and gardens, many of us continue to make fire. Whether in the safety of the stove or wood burner, or outside under the canopies of heaven, this magnetic element has lost none of its appeal.

Whereas homa has very specific instructions – from the construction of the square fire pit, or *kunda*, to the prayers and mantras offered throughout – we've felt inspired by the uplifting practices we've learned from the Vedic tradition, and enjoy sharing little fire rituals with our family, where we set positive intentions and release those things that we wish to move away from, into the cleansing energy of the flames.

---

4   Payne, R., Witzel, M., ed. *Homa Variations: The Study of Ritual Change Across the Longue Durée*; Oxford University Press, 2015, pp. 1–3.

Incense

The *Rig Veda*, the oldest of India's ancient Vedic texts, mentions incense as used during homa rituals. Incense, which was traditionally burned in the form of powder or resin, atop charcoal, was recommended for the clearing of the space – in much the same way that smudging has once again gained popularity.

Alongside resins (such as myrrh, frankincense and pine, all of which are highly purifying) and essential oils that can be made into incense powders or cones, aromatic bark and branches can be added to the fire directly, and burned to clear the space. The most commonly burned wood in Ayurveda is cedarwood, juniper or sagebrush. The incense is quite simply inhaled. In doing so it acts on all layers of the body – physical to energetic. Ayurveda notes that it provides an energetic layer of protection within the space too.

Cleansing with Air

Our little cottage is filled with pairings of naturally air-purifying plants, which clear our space and lift our spirits with their evergreen calm. We began with a plant in each room, but noticed that whenever we placed our peace lilies together, or our dracaena side by side, they perked up immeasurably.

Having since read *The Secret Life of Plants*, we know that plants have their own intimate language and thrive best in families (yes,

#plantshavefeelingstoo). Spider plants, Boston ferns, snake plants, philodendron, Chinese evergreens, lady and bamboo palms are all wonderful for oxygenating and cleansing the home, as they remove carbon dioxide in the day and help to boost oxygen levels.

CLEANSE YOUR BODY

In the West, our emphasis on cleansing often comes with an aggressive undertone, and the modern prevalence for 'detoxing' – whether via spartan juice fasts or out-of-season 'salad' – is wholly anathema to the tender ways in which Ayurveda can support the body to do its own work, painlessly and efficiently, should we so choose.

Indeed, in Ayurveda, the care that we visit upon our body is directly proportional to the health with which it glows. With its inherent quality of unsullied purity of mind and spirit, sattva can be welcomed into daily life via its simple, natural and gentle cleansing rituals.

The Mouth

The Western norm of the plastic toothbrush and synthetic toothpaste is particularly at odds with the Ayurvedic view on oral hygiene. Most commercial toothpastes contain sodium lauryl sulphate – a foaming agent that causes the paste to bubble up and fill the mouth – which has been shown to irritate and dry out skin (and exacerbate mouth ulcers in those who are prone to them.[5]) Many also contain triclosan, a chemical antibacterial that's been prohibited by the US Food and Drug Administration (the FDA) for use in soap and body wash.

Oral hygiene the Ayurvedic way is simpler, and has, hearteningly, been proven to be no less effective in the maintenance of healthy teeth and gums and fresh breath. Ayurvedic tooth powders are sold as powder for a reason – with no water or liquid in the formula, there's no need to add preservatives. Simply wet your toothbrush and coat it with powder. Ayurvedic tooth powders can now be readily purchased online and most contain some or all of the following: cinnamon, ginger, salt, neem, holy basil, sage and clove. If you'd like to make your own, you'll find some lovely suggestions online (we've also shared a recipe at www.thisconsciouslife.co).

Oil Pulling

This much mythologized (though wholly pedestrian) ritual – the simple gargling with oil for some minutes first thing in the morning – has many benefits. While there are many Ayurvedic mouthwashes available (including those that are a mixture of herbs and medicinal oils), most Ayurvedic doctors recommend swilling with cold-pressed organic sesame

---

5   Herlofson, B. B., Barkvoll, P., 1994. 'Sodium lauryl sulfate and recurrent aphthous ulcers. A preliminary study'. www.ncbi.nlm.nih.gov/pubmed/7825393

oil as a gold standard gargle. Sesame is usually a very Pitta-increasing oil, but when gargled with, it's only mildly so. Gargle for long enough for the texture of the oil to change – it should begin to froth and feel thinner in consistency. Three minutes is ample.

While coconut oil is helpful for conditions where Pitta is extremely heightened, it's not as widely recommended for oil pulling as sesame. The benefits of this simple morning ritual are too numerous to list here, but the entire chapter dedicated to this in Acharya Shunya's wonderful book *Ayurveda Lifestyle Wisdom* is a rich resource.

Tongue Scraping

The cleansing of the tongue is another cornerstone of Ayurvedic oral hygiene – you may have heard of 'tongue scraping', which, admittedly, doesn't sound pleasant. Yet this simple, quick and effective ritual is wholly painless. It involves gently drawing a metal instrument down the length of the tongue to clear it of its coating. Tongue scraping quickly makes an enormous difference to the smell, health and function of the mouth – even helping to optimize our sense of taste, as our taste buds are no longer buried beneath a furry residue.

There are many types of tongue scraper available – stainless steel ones are most commonly sold in the West. Ayurveda recommends a gold-plated scraper for tridoshic balancing (which is, of course, expensive), silver-plated for Vata and Pitta balancing, and brass and copper for Pitta and Kapha balancing.

Tongue scraping is always carried out first thing in the morning, after teeth brushing and oil pulling, and before food. It's fine to sip warm water upon waking, but to help your body benefit most from the tongue-scraping process, it makes sense to cleanse the mouth well of the night's accumulated residues before we drink or eat anything significant.

Note: While it can be hard for those who have a particularly sensitive gag reflex to reach to the back of the tongue with their instrument, we've found that doing so slowly and gently, and breathing steadily through the nose at the same time, does help.

Chew Sticks

Traditionally, a chew stick, rather than a toothbrush, is used. These can be sticks taken from the neem, liquorice, guava or arjuna trees (the latter is native to India). While chew sticks are not widely available in the West, they can be ordered online.

Do check which sticks work best with your dosha, and Ayurvedic practitioners also advise against using them when you feel weak, hungover, headachy or thirsty. Made from naturally antibacterial and aromatic woods, they are best seen as a wonderful, purifying addition, rather than a twice-daily tradition.

Dry Powder Massage

Just as dry body brushing – using a bristle brush to stroke the skin from the soles of the feet up to the shoulder blades, before bathing – has become popular in the West, dry powders have equal prominence in Ayurveda.

The act of rubbing the body with dry powders – usually, chickpea or lentil flour is used, mixed with specific herbs for the individual – brings heat to the skin's surface, which is useful in removing toxins, enlivening a sluggish circulation and vitalizing the senses. If skin is more delicate or sensitive, it's recommended that water is added to the powder to make a smooth paste – far less abrasive but still very effective.

Ayurvedic Bathing

Traditionally, one would massage the entire body with warm oil, from the roots of the hair to the soles of the feet, before bathing. The act of stepping into a warm bath, already anointed with oil, is crucial – the skin is then protected from the drying effects of too long an immersion in water: it can be gently cleansed, without harm.

Pages and pages could be written on the various intricate bathing rituals celebrated in Ayurvedic tradition, so significant is bathing's role in physical, spiritual and emotional purification. The main subtext is simple: pleasure. This is a place to retreat, to surrender, to replenish and rebalance.

Ayurveda rarely recommends a cold bath or shower – water should always be warm (it can be hot if Kapha or Vata conditions are heightened). In the height of summer, room temperature water is the lowest you can go: remember, a still, peaceful bath is purest sattva – it's meant to neither overly energize (rajas) nor leave you feeling lethargic (tamas).

At home, we do love a bath. Our children, too, grew up in a home where for a very long time we didn't have a shower. So, filling that tub, anointing the water, sinking beneath it and righting the day's wrongs became part of the natural fabric.

THE AYURVEDIC BATH

Here are some of the things we add to a bath to make it extra special, and beautifully sattvic.

Rose

In Ayurveda, rose is the queen of flowers: it's classified as *hrdya*, meaning 'heart-kind', because of its ability to strengthen our connection with our heart centre. What's good for our heart is good for our whole being, and all those around us – opening us up to an ever-greater capacity to love, and be loved in return. If the week has seemed unkind to you, tempers have frayed and there's been little tolerance for your self and others, rose is your flower.

Rose is revered for its ability to restore the body after extreme fatigue, shock, sadness and grief; at home, we add organic essential oil of rose otto and rosa damascena to our baths – just four or five drops will amply scent the skin and space – and love the ritual of scattering rosebuds (we buy these whole: online or from our beloved local Neal's Yard Remedies) across the surface of the water.

Because they're costly, we scoop them out afterwards, let them dry out and then reuse them. You'd be surprised by how long the scent lingers, so don't automatically discard rosebuds after a single use.

We often pluck the petals from the roses that grow in our little garden, too – fresh velveteen petals feel so lovely against the skin, and if taken from a naturally fragrant variety, release their scent with the steam, making for a delicate, heart-salving soak.

Jasmine

Like rose, which balances all doshas, jasmine is wonderfully restorative. With its heady, 'Arabian Nights' evoking fragrance, a deep lungful and we're transported back to balmy nights in Cyprus. Heaven. In Ayurveda, jasmine is said to be imbued with healing properties that work on imbalances of the eyes, ears and mouth, and it's also useful in the treatment of headaches, heat exposure and sunstroke.

If you don't grow jasmine yourself (it does well in indirect sunlight and shaded areas – coming into full fragrant force under the moonlight), you could invest in jasmine essential oil. Rose and jasmine oils work beautifully together in a bath – balancing all doshas, assuaging fractiousness, dispelling tension and paving the way for a peaceful day, or night.

Calendula

Calendula, also known as 'pot marigold', is a real favourite of ours. For millennia, it's been made into an Ayurvedic salve that's used to help the healing of skin – it's not only supremely gentle, but also naturally antibacterial and antifungal.

From the first year we grew calendula at the allotment, where it flourished and took over a sizeable area, we've not looked back. We harvest and eat it: the petals lend their salubrious properties to stews, soups, porridge and salads (and look beautifully vibrant, scattered atop), where they also balance Pitta and Kapha doshas.

We also dry handfuls of the petals, add them to cold-pressed organic sunflower (tri-doshic) or sesame oil (good for Vata) and infuse for at least a month. You can also strain and add more freshly dried petals to the oil, as many times as you like – each time you'll more potently infuse it (and doing so will give the oil a deeper orange hue). When the oil's ready – and has taken on some of the golden magic of the flowers

– we strain and decant it into dark glass bottles; a litre is enough to keep us in soothing calendula oil for the rest of the year.

We add a good glug of the oil to our baths, or simply scatter the vivid petals into the water directly, where the Ayurvedic benefits really come into their own. Naturally moisturizing, redness-reducing and skin healing, calendula is a beautiful bath-mate (children love the vibrant colour and decorating the sides of the tub with these vivid fronds too).

NATURAL PURIFICATION

The healthy human body purifies itself remarkably well. From our colon, we pass faeces – a natural action that rids us of excess 'earth' (Kapha) and air (Vata). When we urinate, we rid ourselves of excess water, along with the byproducts of our lifestyle – the waste we no longer need; a byproduct of our metabolic processes, uric acid is also cleansed from the blood (Pitta) via the kidneys.

Sweat is linked to the action of the lungs (understood by considering how significantly cardiovascular exercise increases how much we sweat), and this sweat rids us of excess water and toxins we wish to expel. Sweating aids in blood purification (many recent studies on the benefits of infrared saunas have hit our consciousness); it also reduces the fire in the body – naturally cooling us down – and is helpful in the expulsion of excess adipose tissues/fat, which is often where the body holds toxins.

Clearing the Bowel

Seen like this, the 'normal' bodily processes have it covered. When a dosha becomes imbalanced, the body holds the answer in its own inbuilt methods of purification. Ayurvedic doctors tend to agree that one satisfying bowel movement a day (once finished, you feel completely clear, 'empty' and comfortable) is good. This would usually happen in the morning and is helped along by taking the time to rise early, drink warm water upon waking and come into the day slowly – whereby you have the time to expel the previous day's waste before you sit to eat breakfast.

For many of us, however, the morning bowel movement doesn't happen until that first cup of coffee is consumed, or until after breakfast, and if we've had to wake up and rush out of the house before we've properly awoken (physically and mentally), chances are the bowel movement gets pushed back to even later in the day. Or, it simply isn't given a window of opportunity at all.

Clearing the bowel, every morning, is a cornerstone of Ayurvedic health. If we don't 'go' in the morning, the undigested, waste material sits within the body, stored in the bowel – impeding our agni – and the longer it remains, the more it increases in its toxicity. In Ayurveda, the improper function and expulsion of waste from the bowel is seen as the root of many modern diseases. Once, this notion might have been dismissed as impossibly simplistic (and exaggerated), yet today, with our growing knowledge of the gut as the home of good health, we're relearning just how true and far-reaching it really is.

Constipation

All Ayurvedic doctors place a huge amount of importance on bowel movements. Constipation, then, is seen as a digestive disorder that prevents us from feeling wholly healthy and energized. The main causes of constipation are simple – choosing to eat foods that are difficult to digest, in combinations that may not support optimal digestion, at times when we cannot fully digest them; or choosing to eat in ways that preclude our ability to digest well (e.g. grabbing a takeaway breakfast during the rush hour on the way to work, with no bathroom en route to boot).

In the West, we have an obsession with fibre; this is, doubtless, an important part of the nutritional picture, but it's not the panacea for someone who is chronically constipated. The reason is common sense – if you had a blocked drain at home, you wouldn't attempt to clear it with a heavy, dry, rough material. Stuffing yet more 'roughage' into an already blocked pipe will exacerbate the problem. If things are stuck, they need one thing most of all – lubrication.

In Ayurveda, castor oil and aloe vera gel, with their oleating and lubricating qualities, are widely recommended for constipation, as are sesame oil and olive oil; you can take them off a spoon, or simply add them to your meals. Also recommended are teas that help to reignite the digestive fire, and get things 'moving again' – fresh ginger tea is extremely helpful.

Triphala is an Ayurvedic compound that's widely used for chronic constipation (though Dr David Frawley points out that it's not always effective for acute conditions). It can be taken in tablet form, but is traditionally consumed in warm water, before bed. Please check the manufacturer's dosages and instructions, and better still, take a formula that's recommended by a qualified Ayurvedic practitioner.

Note: Because medical advice isn't the remit of this book, we'd advise you to please see an Ayurvedic practitioner (and consult the APA – Ayurvedic Practitioner's Association) before embarking on any Ayurvedic treatment protocol.

Pancha Karma

The most famous, and notorious, of the Ayurvedic cleansing rituals is Pancha Karma, which literally means the five (*pancha*) actions (*karma*). It relates to a rigorous process of purification, carried out under strictest Ayurvedic medical supervision, which brings purity back to the body, mind and spirit.

The five primary actions of pancha karma are *vamana* (therapeutic vomiting), *virechana* (purgation), which encourages multiple bowel movements to thoroughly empty the bowel, *basti* (cleansing enemas), *nasya* (application of cleansing herbs to the nasal passages) and the now mostly outmoded blood-letting, which most Ayurvedic doctors have replaced with blood cleansing, carried out with herbs such as comfrey, turmeric and saffron.

When Pitta is particularly high, there are some who recommend donating blood instead – something we choose to do, partly because we're both quite Pitta in our constitutions, but mostly because we've a real shortage of those in our society who regularly give blood.

We have close friends and colleagues, some of whom are Ayurvedic doctors, who do their annual Pancha Karma as a way to keep their bodies beautifully clear and vital. When there is little ama in the system, pancha karma is more gentle and, often, not all of the five actions are necessary. The approach is always bespoke to the individual – just as you'd hope any medical protocol would be.

All Ayurvedic practitioners are also very clear about the importance of preparing the body in advance of the five actions. *Purva karma*, or pre-actions, should ideally last a full month, during which time one focuses on dosha-specific methods of reducing ama within the body. While we've both lived Ayurvedically for almost a decade now, neither of us has experienced Pancha Karma. If, however, our health threatened to deteriorate or gave us sudden, unforeseen cause for concern, it would doubtless be our first course of action.

Purity Through Fever

Ayurvedic medicine offers some very specific advice on febrile conditions, and the many causes and presentations of different types of fever that may arise from the various imbalances of the doshas. Without going into lots of detail here (there are far more in-depth Ayurvedic medicine and healing books recommended in the Sattvic Resources section), we do feel it's important to talk about what happens to the body when it induces fever.

It's anathema to Ayurveda to seek to suppress any of the body's natural responses – though we can, of course, support it in the work it needs to do. Fever, then, is seen as the body's natural way of purifying itself – and in Ayurvedic medicine, a small dosage of pungent herbs, often imbibed as tea, is used to help the fever run its course more quickly and efficiently.

Fever by Dosha

Much like the fire rituals of the Vedas, we know that fire is incomparably cleansing, and that it leaves behind a literal and figurative clean slate. But what we often see in the West (particularly in young children), is that we develop a fever because our bodies have reached a point of stagnation – agni, our digestive and metabolic fire, may have grown sluggish, which has caused ama, our toxic load, to increase.

In children, this is often seen with the rise in Kapha energy – when the child is producing lots of phlegm and mucous, feels tired and heavy, and clammy or cold to the touch. This is a sign that the body is heavy with dampness, and so it stokes its internal fire in a bid to clear it out as quickly as possible. The hacking cough that often accompanies this state is the result of the body seeking to expel the phlegm that has built up within it.

For Pitta types, fever is restless and irritable. Everything is hot, burning and uncomfortable. Sweating is profuse and can have a sharp smell; likewise, urine is often dark yellow in colour, may sting and can smell acidic.

Vata types often experience achiness and pain in the joints and bones. They will be very restless, and may suffer insomnia during periods of high fever too. It's more common for Vata types to experience constipation during fever, and for their temperature to fluctuate.

Ayurveda recommends that if you can, simply let your fever run its course, making sure to drink plenty of fluids. If you have no appetite, simply sip warm water, thin bone or vegetable broth, or the liquid from a simple homemade soup. It also recommends fresh ginger tea and holy basil (tulsi) tea as wonderful tonics for high fever – they are administered to help the body sweat out its fever, shortening it in the process.

The Ayurvedic herb shatavari (see page 134) is also very useful during instances of low fever – particularly if it has gone on for some time without breaking or clearing. Its tonifying, soothing and hydrating action brings strength back to the tissues, replenishing the inner stores following depletion. Chyavanprash (sometimes called chywanaprash or Golden Preserve in the West) is also a wonderful restorative 'jam' – a traditional Ayurvedic blend of deeply nutritive, balancing herbs and amla fruit, which when taken off the spoon or stirred through warm milk, makes for an excellent tonic for those who have little appetite and low fever.

Ayurveda also considers whether or not the fever coincides with undigested foods in the gut, which have gone on to promote toxins and a build-up of ama (if you've long been constipated, too, and your tongue has a thick white or yellow coating, it could be the root cause). In these instances, it's of primary concern to clear ama and expedite digestion, in which case gentle cleansing herbs such as trikatu, which is also recommended for Vata and Kapha type fevers, are extremely helpful.

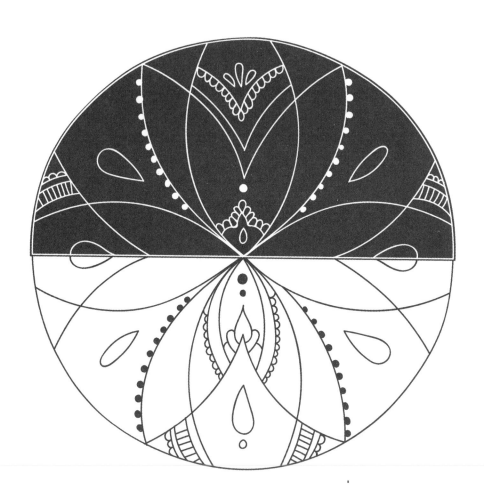

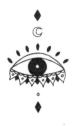

CHAPTER 4

VITALITY

'People subject to ignorance wander to this sacred
place and that sacred place... they do not realize
the sacred place that is within the body.'

JÑANASANKALINI TANTRA

GOOD HEALTH AND VITALITY ARE OUR BIRTHRIGHT. Ayurveda
provides us with a beautifully optimistic picture – one where we
may live richly and well, embracing our selves at every age, thriving
and healthy: a life where good health is the natural result of a sattvic
lifestyle.

Rather than curing illness, Ayurveda seeks to right imbalance at the
outset – to address those early root causes long before they manifest as
unshifting symptoms and chronic conditions. Through sattva we may

move from fear of our mortality and knee-jerk self-medication to the essential joy of life truly lived and loved through each of its seasons.

THREE VITAL ESSENCES

In Ayurveda, there are three vital essences. These are the subtle forms of Vata, Pitta and Kapha, and they exert positive influence over our wellbeing and our vitality:

◊ **Prana**, which we've already discussed, is our vital life force. It's the positive expression of Vata.

◊ **Tejas** is our inner radiance and internal fire (fuelled by Ojas). It sparks our courage, creativity and intellect, and is the positive aspect of Pitta.

◊ **Ojas** is the vital energy of our bodily tissues – our physical vigour and vitality. If we are well nourished and have good digestion and balanced emotions, we have good Ojas.

'A person who has good Ojas rarely becomes sick,' says Dr Vasant Lad, founder of the Ayurvedic Institute. From lustrous hair and healthy skin to a pink tongue and sparkling, bright eyes, we can see Ojas immediately – people look well and we may well comment on it – because it's a lovely thing, and we're programmed to recognize, admire and gravitate towards those who exude good health (evolutionarily, this was, after all, essential when seeking out a viable partner in procreation). 'When Ojas is diminished,' says Dr Lad, 'the person is fearful, weak, and always worried.'

Ojas naturally abounds in children: vital, energetic, clear-skinned, bright-eyed and bushy-tailed – all tissues (dhatus) are strong and function perfectly, from the clear tone of their voice to the pleasing plumpness of their little thighs. This abundant quality – a sense of a beautifully nourished body – is also related to Kapha dosha, which gives us physical resilience and a naturally strong constitution.

Ayurveda believes that if Ojas is strong, we remain well. Dr Vasant Lad describes it as the end product of optimal digestion – all the goodness assimilated from a sattvic diet, paid forward into boundless vitality. Likewise, Ojas flourishes when we live a sattvic lifestyle – choosing softer, slower, more spirit-nourishing activities over those things that numb our senses or overstimulate them. From meditation to Yoga, walks in nature to oil-laced baths – these are the things that encapsulate sattva, and build Ojas in return.

THE THREE LIFE STAGES

Ayurveda teaches us that we have three stages to our human lives, each of which is related to the tri-dosha of Vata-Pitta-Kapha. These are childhood, understood as the period from birth until the age of 16 and a time of Kapha; adulthood, from age 16 to around age 60, which is defined by Pitta, and old age, characterized by Vata from thereon in.

Ayurveda understands the natural human lifespan to be around 100 years, and within this there should only be the beginnings of deterioration when we enter old age. Ayurveda also explains that with excellent Ojas, we can naturally live up to around 120 – those blue-zone centenarians know a great deal about living lives full of sattva, and are all the richer in Ojas as a result. If we live a balanced life, we should remain as vital and active as ever up to the age of 60. This understanding hasn't been adjusted for modern times or modern medicine – it's as it has always been.

Of course, there are many reasons why our physical bodies may not continue to function until the age of 100 (or beyond). The number is a guide as to the rough age at which they naturally break down. The point being, that this breaking down is entirely natural; an attribute of our physical bodies. Those things that are formed of organic matter are finite, and this is the mileage we can expect from our physicality. Death of the body at this point isn't something going wrong, but merely the conclusion of our natural life cycle.

There can be confusion sometimes in our approach to ageing. This lies in whether we're seeking the extension of life at all costs, or whether we're seeking greater health and vitality within it – whether we wish to age gracefully and beautifully, to attain to higher levels of consciousness and to remain happy and active into old age, or whether we're terrified of growing old and dying and nothing short of eternal youth and immortality will do.

If the mind is dominated by tamas, we'll focus on the physical aspects of ageing. We'll rail against each wrinkle, each beautiful silver hair, each sag or dent that tells our stories and ultimately, the dying of the light too. As much as we might try to augment and resculpt, we'll be fighting a losing battle, and it's this fight that's the point here.

Optimal Vitality at Any Age

The sattvic mind acquiesces in and finds beauty in each stage of life. As sattva expands in our minds we naturally move away from body consciousness and towards expansion of the mind and higher, finer energy. This progression flows with the natural movement of our lives – as we grow old we gather wisdom and our physical body naturally fades. This is also the natural course of Yoga, where fear of ageing and death naturally falls away as we attain to higher consciousness.

Sometimes it's important to recognize the distinction between the promotion of life and the prevention of death. Just as health is an active force and not merely the absence of disease, life isn't merely the stuff of not being dead, but a positive state of infinite potential. In our times people are generally longer-lived than our ancestors. As we enter old age and our functioning begins to break down we can now avail ourselves of many means to keep the physical body going – given access to healthcare or the proper insurance – to restore rhythm to a faltering heart, or to change that heart altogether.

More and more drugs are developed and prescribed to address the many symptoms of failing physicality, and then to address the effects of the drugs themselves. Many an old age is spent in a constant adjusting and balancing of diverse pharmaceuticals. This has certainly served to hold death at arm's-length for longer. Whether it promotes *life* is another question. There's little to suggest that we enjoy better health, vitality or enjoyment while we're living than did our ancestors.

Heal Thyself

And sometimes, the opposite is true. Many are experiencing deterioration and disease earlier in life, before they arrive at the stage of old age. In many ways we've outsourced all responsibility for our health and wellbeing to the relevant professionals, and we would have to see many of them to obtain a rounded picture of our holistic health. Our GP will give us a pill for our high blood pressure but isn't well placed to give us comprehensive dietary, lifestyle or environmental advice that's truly individualized – we must go elsewhere for this.

When we're not equipped to make lifestyle adjustments ourselves, or to understand the ways in which we feel and how this relates to our holistic health, we can only rely on professionals and, largely, the treatment of symptoms. Since high blood pressure is a symptom of a deeper imbalance, it will be chemically corrected but the root cause will remain while we continue to take the pill for the rest of our lives.

Before the invention of a pill to lower our dangerously high blood pressure, we had no choice but to seek the necessary lifestyle changes to address the root imbalance or risk facing our mortality.

Ayurveda allows us to take back control of our vitality by equipping us to respond in small ways to the small changes that come with our every day – this is hugely empowering. We find that we can prevent a great deal of ill health before it comes about and more dramatic emergency measures become necessary – requiring further adjustment and recovery. We promote life in a proactive way, rather than reactively staving off disease.

Ayurveda is egalitarian healing. At a time when the impetus of modern science and medicine moves more towards eternal renewal of the healthy and wealthy over healing the sick, and mirrors much of society in this way – and where a great deal of medicine is 'emergency' medicine – Ayurveda can be a great equalizer. Those of us without wealth can prevent sickness and improve our baseline health humbly, naturally, slowly and on our own terms.

THE SATTVIC CHILDHOOD

Children, particularly at a very young age, benefit hugely from an Ayurvedic approach to life – small, preventative, timely adjustments to diet and lifestyle, and little spi-rituals to capture their imagination and further their innate ability to heal and bloom. Modern living, and the disconnection from nature that often accompanies it, hasn't yet disrupted the natural intelligence children carry in their bodies, so they can reap such goodness from intuitive and holistic care and support.

Like adults, nippers have their own unique constitution, their prakriti. Where modern guidance is often a broad brush, understanding your child's prakriti will guide you as to their individual needs and personality traits, and their meanings and revelations.

A child's actual state of balance or imbalance (vikriti), however, is constantly changing; it's shifted slightly by everything: the food they've eaten, the weather, the season, their interactions, activities, impressions, location, sleeping patterns or level of activity. As with adults, they're constantly tipping and redressing, leaning and rebalancing. To learn more about your dosha, your prakriti and your vikriti, visit www.thisconsciouslife.co/discover.

Childhood is a time of Kapha. We can see this in the lustre of our children: their bright eyes, soft, shining skin and the prevalence of Kapha-related imbalances – all the coughs, colds and congestion, particularly in the winter and early spring, where Kapha is seasonally dominant and its heavy, moist and cool nature can be most strongly felt.

Our children crave warmth; they want to be held and enveloped. They are of the body and of the Earth, born into relative inertia and anchored by their nature, physical needs and desires. Kapha is earth, water and solidity and is vital for the rapid bodily development that characterizes childhood. It presides over the nourishment of our tissues, our fat reserves and our balancing of fluids.

Children produce more mucus, which helps to ease the speedy growth of their tissues and protect from dryness and discomfort during this growth. While this time of increased Kapha is essential for physical development, the misery of constant cold-y-ness and the endlessly running nose isn't.

STEPS FOR BALANCING KAPHA IN CHILDREN

We can tune in to our children's unique and shifting natures, as well as those of the season and circumstance, and take small holistic steps to ease the uncomfortable effects of Kapha when it slips out of balance:

- Be aware of the 'qualities' of your child's food, activities and environment. If the moist, oily, cold, heavy and substantive qualities of Kapha are dominant, then meet these with their opposites. For example, food that's light, dry and warm; a warm, dry environment and lively activities to counter the heaviness. Meet your child with your own 'warmth', both physically and through your disposition – this is the real spice of life: magic, lightness and laughter.

- Reduce food of similar quality, such as cold water and dairy products like cold milk and yoghurt; avoid raw, cold or artificially sugary foods, along with overly oily, processed or leftover foods, all of which elevate Kapha. Sweet, sour and salty tastes elevate Kapha too, so try to offer your child balanced meals with a foundation of naturally gentle spice and seasonal veggies (the pungent, astringent and bitter tastes all lower Kapha).

- Reduce the Kapha-elevating effects of milk by using organic milk and serving it warm. Spices such as ginger and cinnamon added to milk will both mitigate Kapha and improve digestion and thereby immunity.

- Fresh, seasonal, cooked vegetables and whole grains will naturally have a warming and drying effect on the body.

- Incorporate spices such as ginger, turmeric, garlic and black pepper into meals.

- Clear and cleanse the nasal passages regularly and rub natural balm or organic sesame oil around the inside of the nostrils. Jal neti (which we explain in the next chapter, Clarity) is excellent for cleansing.

Children: Sattvic Souls

We often focus on what we must teach our children, but rarely consider what we can learn from them. *Vitality*, etymologically and actually, is life – its force and power, its spark or Tejas; its Ojas – fuel and reserves like the wax of a candle – and Prana, the vital flow of energy. Children embody this sattvic quality and we can certainly gather a trick or two from our natural nippers. When we observe our children we should also assume in them a great deal of natural intelligence and look to draw links between their actions and needs.

Childhood is a time of magic, miracle and wonder. This mindset is something to be nurtured rather than educated away. Our memories, and more deeply held events and impressions of childhood, have profound implications for, and power over, our adult lives. Being mindful of your child's sensory world (what they're seeing, hearing, absorbing); their energetic world; the environment in which they live; any unspoken tensions or the hurried or stressed energies we as parents transmit in so many ways, allows us to understand the impressions, associations and qualities of being that will be carried into adulthood.

The doshas are a sideways scale – none is more desirable than the others. Each dosha relates to vital functions and attributes of body and mind, and we seek only to balance them and avoid any becoming unduly raised. The gunas are the 'up and down' – the vertical axis to the doshas' horizontal. Sattvic impressions and associations are nowhere more important and more impactful than during childhood.

Children are already most sattvic souls. Newly born, we have an incredible feeling and experience of connectedness. We don't recognize ourselves as individuals. We don't see where our arm ends and the world begins. We don't discern a difference between us, the people around us and our environment. A newborn baby receives the pure light of pure consciousness. As the brain develops, this is filtered and augmented.

Children are naturally better than grown-ups at being mindful. They more easily lose themselves in the stuff of the moment, focus wholly upon it and create within it. This is an incredibly beneficial tool for alleviating the overwhelming, exhausting impact of the tens of thousands of thoughts we humans think each day – roughly twice as many thoughts as the breaths we breathe – as well as the growing expectations and pace of life culturally imposed on our children.

We have trouble with this when the stuff that captivates them isn't what we'd like them to focus on. When we're trying to get them ready for school, to sit to their breakfast or their homework, to concentrate on dressing themselves, or simply to remain calm and within our eyeline while we complete the work thing we need to finish – we become the nagging distraction – ironically preventing them from being wholly present.

We, in combination with routine, culture and society, condition them away from that time to 'be', observe and evade distraction. Later, when they're grown and stressed, we'll sell it back to them as a little book of mindfulness.

As children begin to crawl, walk, climb, sit, rest and squat, we can observe the staggering intelligence of their bodies. The asana they've mastered without trying – which would take us years of relearning to achieve. If carried into adulthood, the resting and moving postures children adopt with perfect ease would ensure continued flexibility, balance and flow of energy, and protect against degeneration. They have no innate sense of furniture – children are ground-dwelling beings who move, squat, adjust in the most naturally beneficial ways.

This is worth thinking about because it is we who usher them away from this perfection. Biological efficacy doesn't always sit with social conformity, so we sit them in chairs, and tie their eating, their drawing or crafting to the dinner table. We insist on the proper utensils and we put their beautiful bare feet, each with 26 bones, 33 joints and over 100 muscles, ligaments and tendons, into shoes that, slowly but surely, constrict the spread of their toes, affect their natural movement and subtly alter the whole of their posture from the ground up.

Love Without Condition

Our children are subject to many diverse pieces of information to which they are much more open than us adults, who are already heavily conditioned in one direction or another (or many) by our own formative years.

While children have the capacity to play wildly imaginative games for hours on end, using nothing but a stick, a pile of pebbles, a cardboard box, a swatch of woodland or just one another, they're often also infiltrated from an early age by the cultural and economic belief that they must amass possessions, and that their 'value' is directly related to this. Higher, sattvic play, which begins in the imagination and emanates from the mind, is slowly replaced by a tamasic rooting of worth and enjoyment in the physical and material.

Children crave our unconditional love and our dedicated time. They are happily furnished with energy, time and spirit of adventure in abundance. Grown-ups, however, often lack these. We'll speak more of prevailing culture in the final chapter, but children often receive conditional gifts in place of the unconditional love they really need. They often receive distraction and entertainment, such as television, toys and computer games, in place of our attention. They then join the dots and begin to equate possessions and distractions with love and time.

They understand their worth in these terms: 'I was really good today so Daddy bought me some sweets and let me watch a movie.' 'Grandma bought me the biggest toy in the shop, so she must love me very much.' Later, if these things are denied, then 'love' itself is being withdrawn.

As children develop, this is what they understand of love. Processed foodstuffs of no real nutritional value, sweets and stimulants, toys made out of plastic. Things to own and electronic entertainment are all spuriously elevated – a measure of what your beautiful, natural child is worth and their 'success' in doing what's expected of them. When they're older, they're likely to overindulge in these things because they've been sanctified. They sit on a pedestal with the dusty legend: 'My parents' time and devotion.' And they're likely to 'love' their own children by the same means.

The actual narrative can run more like, 'Daddy didn't have the time or energy to spend with me dedicatedly – he had an important email and a report to finish – so he gave me some sweets and turned on the TV to keep me occupied.' 'Grandma hasn't been around much and feels bad about it, so she bought me the biggest toy in the shop.'

Busy guardians pacify their children because real sattvic nourishment takes real time, real energy and real presence, in the moment, and on the child's own terms. We create fictional subtexts because the reality runs counter to our own natural instincts and intuition as parents and nurturers. It's hard to admit that we simply didn't find the time or energy for our child; it's easier and more comfortable to convince ourselves that we had their best interests at heart or wanted to 'treat' them. We should be honest about these things because children will truly take us at our word – the seeds sown in childhood are deeply planted, and they will grow and bear fruit.

WAYS TO SAVOUR SATTVA IN CHILDHOOD

- Join your children in stories and magic; in their links to nature and the elements. Play with them in the woods, tell stories collectively around the campfire – allow them to lead you in play while you avoid 'correcting' and 'teaching'.

- Allow a full sensory experience around food. Try eating meals on the ground, at a low table, and watch their movement and posture; allow them to use their hands, and provide a variety of ingredients for them to control – toasted seeds or various herbs to scatter, oils to dress or citrus to squeeze over their food. Support them to grow, gather and cook with you – nurture their relationship with, and enjoyment of, food.

- Help children to avoid too much artificial stimulation. Turn all screens off in the mornings and at least an hour before sleep. Encourage them away from the chairs and sofas and onto the floor – try soft rugs or cushions (they're comfortable there!) Help them to experience and absorb sattvic impressions:

pleasant, natural sights, sounds and scents; natural light, fresh air and time spent outdoors in natural settings – to run, climb, play and immerse themselves in all the rhythms and textures.

- Try to be slow and allow children to become lost in the natural, non-electronic, things that captivate them. Allow them to stare out of the window, to observe or to do nothing at all. We don't have to distract constantly, fill every moment with substance or rush them from club to club.

- Remember that their life is already happening and isn't only to be spent in preparation for a somehow more 'real' life when they're fully grown. Mindfulness and stillness are excellent tools for the whole of our lives. This is difficult when we're school- and work-running, but balancing the pace of our lives culturally with periods of slow is essential in growing sattva.

- Give unconditional love and constant reminders of this love. Avoid a continued cycle of punishment and reward and be mindful of the 'treats' you're offering, as these will be elevated in the mind of your child.

- Avoid violence, even where you admonish your child's actions. Don't shout or lose your temper. Admit your own mistakes, limitations and moods. If consequences must be put in place, do this gently and balance with reiteration of your unconditional love. A punishment isn't a withdrawal of love. A reward isn't greater love bestowed. Love is constant. There is great safety and comfort in this.

AYURVEDIC HERBAL MEDICINE

Dravya-guna Shastra, the Ayurvedic science of medical substances, literally means the science (*shastra*) of substances (*dravya*) and their qualities (*guna*). It's a vast and fascinating subject, and we're going to touch on it, most gently, here (we recommend Dr David Frawley's *The Yoga of Herbs* as a wonderful follow-on, if this area is of particular interest to you).

Because herbal medicine in accordance with Ayurveda focuses on the gunas of plants, we find a beautifully illuminating road map that helps us to identify things that will support us in raising our sattva – as many Ayurvedic herbs do so naturally. There are also herbs that have a heightened enlivening effect (rajas) or dulling effect (tamas).

Aside from the naturally vitalizing antioxidant benefits of Ayurvedic herbs, which help to bolster our bodies against the day's natural (and unnatural) wear and tear, many Ayurvedic herbs also possess remarkable '360' qualities – shown to help with myriad different conditions and proven to have benefits across mind, body and spirit.

At first, it may seem unlikely that a herb proven to speed the healing of wounds has also been shown to reduce the symptoms of anxiety. In the West, this can trigger our cynicism; we're used to the black-and-white prescription and the taking of a single tablet for a single symptom.

But in Ayurveda, as we've already amply explored, we're not divisible fragments, we're made to be whole. And when we accept this idea, we might begin to see how it makes even more sense to assume, for example, that a natural medicine that helps to bolster our gut health, might also promote positive mental health (something that modern science now supports, with an estimated 70 per cent of our happy hormone, serotonin, known to be made in the lining of the gut).

NATURAL VERSUS SYNTHETIC MEDICINE

Interestingly, all 'drugs', i.e. inorganic synthetic medicines, are viewed as tamas by Ayurveda because they're heavy and unnatural. This entire process is one that works to dull the senses and has long-term desensitizing effects.

Synthetic drugs can also suppress our natural immune response: we may rush to take paracetamol to bring down a fever, but today we're relearning the importance of letting the fever run its course, with a raft of recent studies proving that much of the time, intervening isn't particularly helpful and can, on occasion, do more harm than good.[6] Although there are, of course, exceptions, particularly in infancy, when utmost caution is always recommended.

---

6   Ray, J. J., and Schulman, C, I., 2015. 'Fever: suppress or let it ride?' www.ncbi.nlm.nih.gov/pmc/articles/
    PMC4703655

One painkiller can provide relief but continual usage dulls our sensory mechanisms – we become so reliant on pain relief that we lose sight of what a natural physical response to pain might be (and most crushingly, what is really at the root cause of that pain in the first place).

Commercial pharmaceuticals are also mass-produced in leviathan quantities, in a way that consumes a huge amount of energy and can produce a great deal of heat. This is anathema to the production of Ayurvedic herbal medicines, which are traditionally made by hand, for the individual, in tiny batches, and administered fresh.

Ayurvedic Medicine

While many Ayurvedic herbs are now widely available in tablet form, and sold worldwide in increasingly large quantities, it's also important to seek to understand how they are grown and where, by whom they are harvested, and whether or not the indigenous herb itself is being taxed or depleted by this cultivation.

Sadly, many traditional Ayurvedic herbs are becoming increasingly endangered – perhaps given our growing appetite for and awareness of Ayurveda, we, too, are to blame. Again, conscious choices need to be made. The answer isn't always complicated. Often, the herb we seek to import from distant, tropical climes is rivalled in its benefits by the one that grows just metres from our own doorstep.

The more we learn about herbs, the more we realize this too. The incredible goosegrass, nettle, rosemary, thyme, oregano, parsley and mint possess many impressive properties, and at home, we seek to balance those things we source ethically from far-flung places with the dozen we now grow in the land upon which we live, or those to be found on a wild country walk.

Gut health

Looking after your child's digestion and the health of the rich and delicate bacterial balance in the gut is of huge importance too. This is the main source of their immunity, and where they obtain and assimilate their nourishment. Numerous studies have confirmed that babies who are born vaginally have the immunity advantage – exposure to the vaginal microflora during delivery leads to the normal microbial 'seeding' of the baby's gastrointestinal tract; the baby's virgin digestive system is literally lined from the mouth down with their mother's unique strains of complex bacteria, which gives them a measurable head start in the good bacteria stakes.[7]

For Ayurveda, it's always been simple – the strength of our gut, our digestive fire, our agni is one of the most accurate markers of good health that we have, and the ripple effects of what we consume and imbibe are felt not only in the stomach, but also by the whole of us – a terrible stomach ache or acid reflux will of course affect our mood and

---

7   Neu, J., and Rushing, J., 2012. 'Cesarean versus Vaginal Delivery: Long term infant outcomes and the Hygiene Hypothesis'. www.ncbi.nlm.nih.gov/pmc/articles/PMC3110651

overall sense of wellbeing. Allopathy may focus solely on a substance's action at a physical level, but in Ayurveda, we recognize the subtle and energetic responses too. All is connected, and so that's how we choose to approach our health – always, and in all ways.

Using Herbs at Home

There are many Ayurvedic herbs that can be grown in the house or garden. For those who don't have the means, time or space to do so, though, many are available in dried, powdered or supplement form, and as teas – all of which have their useful spot and purpose in our sattvic home.

Many Ayurvedic herbs are naturally adaptogenic. Adaptogens possess a unique combination of pharmacological actions which, when absorbed by the body, help it adapt to its stressors, promoting better health and resilience. Many are also incredibly high in antioxidant properties, which means that they have the ability to mop up the free radicals that cause oxidation and oxidative stress.

This natural detoxification is incredibly useful when we consider the rising levels of pollution and electromagnetic and chemical interference we're being subjected to. This is Mother Nature's way of fighting back and enabling us to thrive too – even if humankind can sometimes seem blindly and blithely set on self-destruction.

In Ayurveda, however, the use of herbs only ever works in conjunction with the Ayurvedic diet and Ayurvedic lifestyle. It's not a standalone approach. All Ayurvedic doctors believe that the body can be brought into happy balance if one is eating in tune with one's own bodily constitution and needs – that food builds the body and that herbs help to correct its subtle physical imbalances.

Also of primary importance is honouring your own doshic predisposition (your innate constitution, or prakriti; see page 40) and living in a way that supports, rather than aggravates, your strengths and weaknesses. It's all very well taking a mind-calming tonic for stress, but if you refuse to go to bed, turn off your phone, slow down, relax or eat good food, it won't even touch the sides. There's no pill, Ayurvedic or otherwise, that will counterbalance a life built on bad choices.

Ayurveda is forgiving and pragmatic: if you're accustomed to drinking alcohol heavily and are reluctant to reduce the amount, an Ayurvedic doctor might suggest that you vary what you drink, and choose drinks of better quality. Drinks can be chosen according to dosha and imbalance, and preparations or herbal packs to bolster the liver may be administered. Ultimately, though, 'make better choices' would be their matter-of-fact advice, along with, perhaps, a truthful: 'What do you expect to feel if you live this way?' Who can argue with that?

With diet and lifestyle taken care of, however, herbs are seen to be incredibly useful. The premise is simple – all things in nature can benefit us, if they're used correctly. We often share our stories of our time in the biodynamic gardens at Weleda – a company that produces natural beauty and wellbeing products alongside naturopathic medicines – where plants such as rhus tox (poison ivy), aconite, henbane and belladonna can be irritating and venomous in their raw state but are well-used in homeopathic healing.

Again, it's the dose that makes the poison. It's never recommended that you take herbs alone to remedy your ills, but as an extra layer of balancing and bolstering support, they can be truly remarkable.

Tulsi

Tulsi, or holy basil, is one of Ayurveda's most important plants, reverently named 'the queen of herbs'. Its well-researched benefits[8] are too extensive to fully explore here, but this natural adaptogen is a herb that we like to have close to hand. Modern studies have repeatedly found that tulsi possesses notable anti-anxiety and antidepressant properties.[9]

---

8   Cohen, M. M., 2014. 'Tulsi - *Ocimum sanctum*: A herb for all reasons'. www.ncbi.nlm.nih.gov/pmc/articles/PMC4296439

---

9   Bhattacharyya, D. et al, 2008. 'Controlled programmed trial of *Ocimum sanctum* leaf on generalized anxiety disorders'. www.ncbi.nlm.nih.gov/pubmed/19253862

Its unique broad-spectrum benefits also include antibacterial, antioxidant, anti-inflammatory and analgesic actions.

Excitingly, too, tulsi increases the body's levels of some very helpful antioxidant molecules, such as glutathione, and enhances the efficacy of our natural antioxidant enzymes, such as superoxide dismutase – wonderful moppers-up of free radicals and chemical toxins.[10] Available in plant form, this short-lived perennial can be very easily grown in pots and is resilient to most weather conditions. The fresh leaves can be steeped in hot water to make tulsi tea – a mild and pleasant tonic with a soothing scent that belies its bountiful benefits. You can also buy tulsi tea ever more widely, or find it in powdered form, which is useful if mixing with liquid or milk.

Brahmi
....

Knowing that the word *brahmi* is taken from the Sanskrit *brahman*, 'the totality of life', we can begin to imagine the significance of this holiest of Ayurvedic herbs, which is also said to be a potent mind-expander and a route to higher consciousness. It's ironic, then, that the name of this herb continues to provoke debate.

In South India, brahmi most often relates to bacopa, or water hyssop (latin name, *Baccopa monnieri*), whereas in North India, brahmi most often

---

10　Shivananjappa M., Joshi M. 'Aqueous extract of tulsi enhances endogenous antioxidant defenses of human hepatoma cell line (HepG2)', *J Herbs Spices Med Plants*, 2012; 18:331–48.

refers to gotu kola (latin name, *Centella asiatica*). This duality has arisen from the fact that in ancient times, both bacopa and centella were most commonly used together, and it was this combination of herbs that was referred to as 'brahmi'.

Brahmi was traditionally used to help sharpen concentration during lengthy periods of hymn recital and learning, and is lauded as the most sattvic of all herbs, for its ability to promote tranquillity and peace of mind.

And, just as brahmi is valued for its mind-cleansing properties, it's equally lauded for its purifying attributes. With both a bitter and astringent taste, it's a wonderful tonic for excess toxins, or ama, encouraging the body to cleanse and clear toxins from the tissues in much the same way that it promotes the release of negative thoughts from the mind. Brahmi is also said to raise Ojas – the body's vigour and vitality – and from a Western viewpoint, its tonifying effect on the nervous system is well researched too. Bacopa is widely sold in plant form; it's a hardy perennial, which means it will thrive in most conditions for up to three years.

Gotu kola (centella) is also useful when making medicated butters (where herbs are cooked with ghee to form a potent herbal remedy). This is best done under the guidance of an Ayurvedic practitioner, or you can buy medicated butters online from reputable Ayurvedic suppliers.

Ashwagandha

In recent years, we've seen the rise in awareness and popularity of this most powerful and helpful Ayurvedic herb. It's been hailed as a cure-all for modern life's myriad ills and, refreshingly, the hype is real – but there is the odd caveat to be aware of.

Ashwagandha, also known as Indian ginseng or Indian winter cherry, is incredibly useful for many things. *Ashwa* means horse, and so it's said that the intelligent consumption of this herb bestows upon us the strength of one. As an adaptogen, it's used as a rejuvenative (rasayana), whereby it promotes a stronger constitution and more resilient mind – aiding the body in better coping with psychological and physiological stress. It's particularly helpful as a nervine tonic because of its dual ability to promote both vitality and calmness, at the same time.

If this seems odd, consider that the ideal state is when we're full of purpose and natural, balanced energy, while still feeling calm and in control. Ashwagandha helps us here. It has been shown to be helpful in the prevention of neurodegenerative diseases such as Alzheimer's, Parkinson's and Huntington's,[11] and as effective protection against gastric ulcers caused by aspirin or stress-related conditions.[12]

---

11   Singh, N. et al, 2011. 'An Overview on Ashwagandha: A Rasayana (Rejuvenator) of Ayurveda'. www.ncbi. nlm.nih.gov/pmc/articles/PMC3252722

---

12   Singh, N. et al. *'Withania Somnifera* (Ashwagandha), a Rejuvenator Herbal Drug Which Enhances Survival During Stress (an Adaptogen)'. *Int J Crude Drug Res.* 1982; 3:29–35.

Ashwagandha has also been shown to be helpful in the management of mood disorders, including anxiety and depression. It does, however, raise Pitta in the body, so it's not recommended for those individuals whose Pitta is already elevated. Likewise, if the body is already carrying excessive ama, caution is advised. It is, in general terms, wonderful for balancing Vata and Kapha.

Shatavari

Known as the women's herb, shatavari literally means 100 (*shat*) roots (*vari*). Vari can also mean husband, leading us a little closer to this asparagus-like root's phallic significance – giving it the nickname 'she of 100 husbands'. It's a wonderful rejuvenative for all women and purest sattva in its quality – not only calming and balancing, but also heightening our capacity to feel love and devotion.[13]

Shatavari has always been used to beautiful effect in the promotion of overall fertility and a smoother menstrual cycle with regulated mood; it's been studied as a breastfeeding aid, too, where it was shown to significantly improve the release of prolactin in lactating mothers.[14]

---

13   Frawley, D., Lad, V., 2001. *The Yoga of Herbs: An Ayurvedic Guide to Herbal Medicine*, Lotus Press.

14   Gupta, M. and Shaw, B., 2011. 'A Double-Blind Randomized Clinical Trial for Evaluation of Galactogogue Activity of *Asparagus racemosus* Willd'. www.ncbi.nlm.nih.gov/pmc/articles/PMC3869575

It's also a wonderful balancing and bolstering herb for the female body during menopause (and for those women who have had a hysterectomy), as it's been shown to possess phyto-oestrogenic properties (a plant source rich in natural oestrogen).[15] For peace of mind, alongside body, there are also no known contraindications or negative interactions with hormonal medication, such as the contraceptive pill or HRT.

---

15   Ashajyothi, V., 2009. '*Asparagus racemosus* – a Phytoestrogen'. www.researchgate.net/publication/44024760

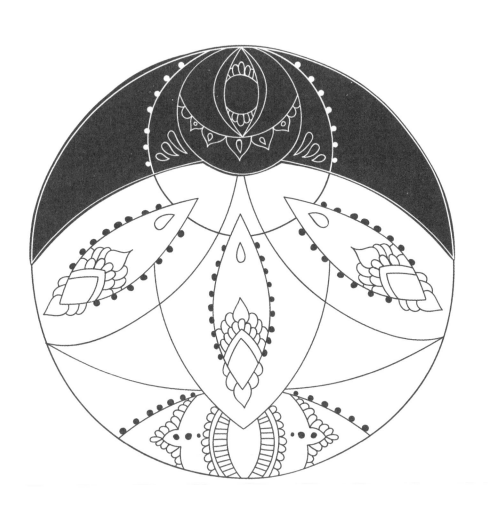

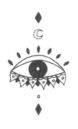

CHAPTER 5

CLARITY

'Unless the mind is calm and clear, we cannot
perceive anything properly. Sattva creates clarity,
through which we perceive the truth of things.'

DR DAVID FRAWLEY,
AYURVEDA AND THE MIND: THE HEALING OF CONSCIOUSNESS

WE DON'T ONLY EXPERIENCE THE WORLD THROUGH OUR SENSES, we enter it according to our level of consciousness and we avoid it according to our past experiences. Through the noise of our thoughts, desires and surroundings, or the limitations and changeability of our perception, our awareness can be obscured, clouded and augmented.

We may view an identical scenario quite differently on different days – based on nothing more than the amount of sleep we've had, what we've eaten, or what conversation preceded it. We can, all of us at times, feel like four seasons in one day. But through sattvic practice, we can choose not just our own identity, but the truth of the world around us – becoming increasingly aware of how it's not, in fact, the facts presented that affect us, but how we choose to respond to them, that counts.

CULTIVATE POSITIVITY

It can be beautiful to throw open our senses to the world, especially in nature – perhaps walking in the woods or lying on the grass with no agenda. Here we can live in that right-brained flood of natural information and allow all the healing subtleties of birdsong, breeze and buzz to wash over and through us. This was the daily meditation of our hunter-gatherer ancestors: to be in nature, fully open and receptive to the deep osmosis of shared resonance.

In Vedic science the impressions and information we receive are part of our *food* (*ahara*); they combine with our being and, just like the food we eat, can be both nourishing and damaging. In the spirit of being gentle on ourselves we should never grasp or suppress these impressions; however, it's essential, particularly when we return from the woods or the grassland to the 'real world', to accept and consciously embrace those that are healing, sustaining and pleasing, and allow darker, more upsetting information to roll and rise like steam from our being.

By 'upsetting' we mean in the context of an apple cart or a bucket – which tips the balance and prevents us from rolling along the road or erodes our capacity to receive and contain. There are dark aspects to every person's reality. There are daily disappointments, unpleasant images, places, scents and scenes through which we must sometimes walk. There are tragedies, heart-rending occurrences and unfairnesses every day, globally and locally: on the front page (though often closer to the back), in our homes and those of our neighbours.

At these times it's natural to feel deep empathy and to share in the experience of others – that which frightens, haunts and hurts them. If, however, we're laid low by these or allow hurtful impressions to adhere collectively to our being, we upset our own balance of light and dark and are prevented from being the helping hand or guiding torch that might help to relieve the suffering of others.

This isn't about being blithe or sticking our fingers in our ears, 'la, la, la… can't hear you'. Just as our reasoning is impaired when we're angry or stressed, so, too, is our capacity for compassion and positive action.

As we've said, stress is the shutting down of non-vital functioning in order to flee or fight. When we feel outraged or deeply sad, we can often lash out into negativity, rather than seek the positive action or advice that will improve the situation. This can be seen every day, when our 'upset' at a particular global unfairness that enters our awareness is translated into hatred, anger or vengeful thoughts towards the corporation, government, official, faction or religion we deem responsible.

It can also be seen more simply when a fellow driver forces us into a pothole or presents us with the finger and we carry and replay the residual anger throughout the day – foisting it on the next unfortunate driver to come along, or scolding our children unnecessarily. Those around us will pass our anger along and together we spread the dark and block the light. It's not weakness to let something go. It's purest strength – to rise above. There is such peace above the clouds.

True clarity is found in understanding that there will be many actions, images and impressions arriving via our senses that carry a negative colour or charge, but resolving that these won't throw us from our path or prevent us from treating all other beings with compassion. As self-care helps us to find the reserves we need to care for others, cultivating positivity will allow others to feel positive too. And there's that win-win again.

FEED YOUR SPIRIT

The yogic practice of *Pratyahara* is sometimes understood as simply withdrawal from the senses and shifting our attention inwards, but it's much more than this. It's conscious governance of our sensory 'food' – choosing to control the external things that can damage our cups and leave us with a vessel from which we cannot pour. It's not covering our eyes, like the first of those little monkeys; it's seeing not 'evil', but imbalance, trauma and negativity in others and refusing, slowly but surely, to be its conduit or keeper.

One meaning of the Sanskrit word *samskara* is a stain on our spiritual fabric, or a wound that we carry from our past actions. Action (karma) begins with intention, and a samskara is the subtle mark made on our being that carries the intention and thereby the impetus behind, and power of, our actions. Over our lifetimes our nervous systems will carry many such stains, each a smudge on the glass through which we view or reflect the world. Sattva, on the other hand, is clear-sightedness: impervious to all that our senses can bombard us with.

Bright Eyes

Ayurveda and Yoga promote clarity in various physical ways that flow from the senses to the spirit. A good example of this is *trataka* or candle meditation. Regular trataka practice promotes eye health through cleansing – improving and refining vision. It's also a beautiful, lulling meditative practice to help soothe a restless mind and alleviate anxiety.

Trataka doesn't involve staring into a flickering flame, as is sometimes thought. A flickering candle reflects a rajasic mind – darting, dancing, never still – and for trataka the flame should always be still. For this you need a darkened space free of draughts and breezes. It's recommended that trataka be first learned through guided practice and, given the sensitivity of the eyes, we think so too, so we haven't described the technique in full here.

Trataka involves gently moving the gaze in very specific ways, from the candle base to the flame and around the aspects of the room or space, closing and resting the eyes intermittently and applying the eyes' attention to the different layers and qualities of the flame. Seeking qualified instruction from a yogic practitioner, and establishing a regular practice, is a great way to nurture the connection between ocular clarity and the clarity of the mind in stillness; to soften anxious impulses and keep eyes bright.

PRANAYAMA FOR CLARITY
– THE HEAD CLEARING BREATH

Kapala bhati is an excellent pranayama for restoring clarity: it's like that well-needed strong shot of coffee – perfect for the mid-morning dip, or that 4 p.m. drowsiness, but without the jitters or the lull that can follow. In Sanskrit, kapal means skull and bhati means shining – the breath for a clear, illuminated mind. Kapala bhati can be practised in the time it takes to sink a cup of the black stuff and, rather than feeling wired, it will leave you feeling peaceful, renewed and receptive.

It also improves respiration by invigorating the lungs and respiratory tract. Let's begin:

1. Sit comfortably, either cross-legged on the floor or in a chair, keeping your neck and spine upright.

2. Close your eyes and be still for a moment, holding your right hand to your abdomen.

3. Focus on your exhalation and breathe rapidly through your nose – two exhalations to each second. Your exhalation should be forceful, the inhalation automatic.

4. With your right hand, feel your abdomen contract with each exhalation.

5. Breathe in this way for one minute.

As you stop the practice you'll feel a stillness come over you and your breathing will stop entirely for a few seconds – a beautiful sense of peace after which you'll feel energized and restored.

Nasal Cleansing

The simplest actions, rooted in hygiene, can be deeply spiritual acts. Ayurveda advises many such cleansing processes, and the freeing and opening of our bodily and energetic channels, both to alleviate bodily pressures and imbalance in our daily lives, and as preparation for higher practice such as meditation, which is greatly enhanced by the free flow of our breath and Prana.

Many things pervade our nostrils every day: in the classroom, at the road or fireside, in a pollen-rich meadow or dusty track. Cleansing our sinuses improves our olfactory capacity, draws excessive heat from the brain and can help to prevent headaches, sinusitis, migraine, hay fever, inflammation and infection, and improve symptoms of asthma. Most strikingly, it brings relief and free flow.

JAL NETI

This simple ritual to maintain nasal clarity requires only a 'neti pot' – a small pot with a long, narrow spout – warm water and salt. A copper neti pot is best. A sitting position helps with jal neti – perhaps outside – but you can also do it standing over a sink:

- Add one teaspoon of sea salt to 500 ml (just under a pint) of purified warm water (water boiled, then cooled to warm is fine) and pour it into the pot. Then place the cone at the end of the spout inside the right nostril.

- Breathing through your open mouth, tilt your head gently to the left and slightly forwards, and adjust until the water begins to flow from the left nostril. (This can feel quite strange to begin with and you may sneeze or cough, but regular practice will bring ease as you find the correct positioning.) Allow all of the water in the pot to flow from the left nostril.

· Refill the pot and repeat, this time placing the cone into the left nostril and allowing it to flow through the right nostril.

· It's very important to make sure that your nose feels empty and dry following jal neti. Practise kapala bhati – see above – to remove excess moisture from the nasal cavity, and dry with a cloth or towel. Once dry, applying a drop of sesame oil, rubbed around the inside of the nostril, will ease any irritation and help to maintain clarity.

Making Light

Cultivating positive impressions and seeking the lighter side of a given situation helps to bring balance to our being. An experience or event is something we carry with us, stored like data in our nervous system. We've evolved to hold on to negative experiences, and we archive these for future reference so that traumatic events aren't repeated. We'll feel this when we experience an intuitive block towards a particular situation, or perhaps an opportunity.

Subconsciously, we've flagged these as being related to past trauma. When we have a build-up of these negative associations we become blocked in many directions. Even if, in a rational or intellectual sense, we've learned from or resolved past issues, many of our actions can feel difficult, stress-inducing or counterintuitive.

We may dread having to approach certain situations, without understanding why, since the associations from which these blocks are derived are deeply entombed in our subconscious and cannot be exhumed by our rationality or willpower alone. These may be simple and everyday situations relating to our work, travel or family. Telling ourselves to 'snap out of it', or simply pushing through anxiety and stress can be exhausting and lead us into further negative experience. The scope of our lives begins to shrink and close; our vision pervaded by subtle, peripheral shadows and accompanied by the narrowing of our potential.

It's not so difficult to understand and relate to these feelings and the shrinking of our world as we grow older and accumulate these impressions. Contrast your adult experience with that as a wide-eyed child: open, eager and fearless. Or earlier, as a newly born baby, where all things were an inextricable, oceanic extension of yourself and you knew only trust.

It's deeply liberating and rejuvenating when we may steadily resolve and remove these blocks, meeting them at the deepest, most subtle levels and gently and easily let them go. When we do this, we begin to widen, rather than narrow, our vision and clarity. We expand our potential and we open ourselves to experience and all the wonderful stuff of life. We don't have to overcome anxiety and fear. We can just remove the conditions for their residence within us.

Meditation for Clarity

As mentioned earlier, we both sit to practise Vedic meditation once, ideally twice, a day. When we learned Vedic meditation, we were each given our own mantra by our teacher. This mantra is an energized sound – a sacred word – that's chanted repeatedly in the mind: a point to return to each time other thoughts rise up and interrupt, as they naturally will.

By returning to the mantra in our minds, we disempower all of those thousands of extraneous and unhelpful thoughts that can very easily take over our headspace. The purpose of meditation is to support the mind in its natural pursuit of bliss – a direction that brings about ever-deeper physical and mental rest, and healing. The sensation of sitting in meditation with one's mantra is of a cosmic whisper, guiding us back, comforting, lifting, clearing – immensely soothing and powerful.

As we meditate, thoughts continue to cascade in and rise up – of course they do, and always will – but the repeated mantra presides and allows the mind to follow its natural direction. So, instead of running away with a thought (*I forgot to make that call! The world will come to an end!*), thoughts surface like bubbles of release as we continue to repeat our mantra effortlessly. Perspective is restored, the mind is refreshed and recharged, and we're relieved of the never-ending cycle of reactive thoughts.

The results of numerous robust, research-led studies into Vedic meditation – which is related closely to transcendental meditation – are extraordinarily clear. Our meditation teacher Will Williams says: 'When we meditate, we rest three to five times deeper than the deepest part of sleep. It enables us to repair so deeply that all of these distortions start to unwind and re-calibrate towards normal functioning again.' Vedic meditation also immediately decreases the production of the stress hormone cortisol by an average of 33 per cent.

Gentle Self-Awareness

Dr David Frawley says, 'Unless we learn to look within, we will remain trapped in the outer mind and not know how to penetrate through the core of ignorance within us. Only when in contact with our Inner Self can we unlock the secrets of awareness.'

Awareness is the most precious gift that we can give to our self. It allows us to make wise and helpful decisions as we move through our lives. It allows us to step back and realize that we no longer want to smoke 20 cigarettes a day or fall into bed at 2 a.m. every night; that those remnants of our past are outdated and unhelpful and we may choose to leave them behind.

Awareness helps us to shift our habits towards those that will nourish our selves, inside and out, because we're making conscious choices that benefit the whole of our being. Our tremendous innate capacity for healing isn't limited to the physical wear and tear that we experience. To heal deeply, mentally, spiritually we don't need to push, strain or even actively seek it. We only need to allow it. For this, we need only clarity.

YOU ARE MULTITUDES

As our need for healing doesn't live only in the tamas of the physical, nor do we. We're not only physical beings but also energetic beings, capable of straddling different layers of consciousness and formed of our deeply embedded impressions.

In describing this, Ayurveda recognizes the body in ways that are separate to the *physical*, or *gross* body. We have our *subtle* or *energetic* body – created through all that we feel and experience via our senses and thoughts, and the cycling of our natural energy. We have our *causal* body, made of impressions, which is where we hold our most deeply rooted nature. We use our physical body when we're awake, our subtle body when we dream, and only ever experience our causal body when we're in deepest sleep or profoundest, transcendent meditation.

The Five Layers of Self

Ayurveda provides a clear overview on how we can 'inhabit' our three bodies – physically, energetically and spiritually – and further stratifies them into the *panchakosha*: the five sheaths or layers of self. This is the scale of ever finer, higher and more subtle energy that comprises our whole being and consciousness.

Annamaya Kosha

Our physical layer of flesh and bone, skin, sinew and viscera; *annamaya kosha* takes in material food and eliminates material waste.

Pranamaya Kosha

This layer is formed of our vital energy, or Prana, and includes our breath; it's our vitality, which flows into and out of our bodies.

Manomaya Kosha or Manas

This layer comprises the mind and all that relates to our thoughts and ego (*ahamkara*). It's the 'I' and the 'Me'; our individualism. The 'me' we perceive, however, expresses itself in language and associations taken from our conditioning and society. However 'personal' we believe it to be, it's derived of aspects that are not 'self'-generated.

Vijnanamaya Kosha

Our body of intelligence, or *buddhi*, *vijnanamaya kosha* is our intellect, reason and the space where we perceive, discern, discriminate, will or form intention. It's the font of enlightenment and truth. We aim to develop buddhi as our body of higher intelligence and to diminish our body of mental distraction or disturbance (*chitta*). It can be easy to imagine that the reasoning and discrimination we commonly understand as human consciousness is our true or higher self. However, this sheath of being is changeable, endowed with limits and, crucially, not always there.

Anandamaya Kosha

This is the state of bliss (*ananda*) and is linked inextricably to the causal body. *Anandamaya kosha* is our innermost 'self' (*atman*), pure, unfiltered consciousness and the ultimate direction of spiritual practice and meditation. When our minds and senses rest as in deepest sleep, outside of both waking and dreaming, it's the self that remains and ties us to the world we know.

Here we are free of all desire and attachment, fear, anxiety and suffering. Here we find our highest, most healing and subtle brain states, our deepest rest and our greatest sense of connection. It's where our minds will go if we allow them. Vedic meditation facilitates the mind in its natural pursuit of bliss, and with it comes ever-increasing empathy, compassion, calm and clarity.

We find it really comforting and illuminating to think of our selves in terms of all of the various physical, spiritual and psychological 'parts'. Not just because it goes some way to explaining just how complex we really are and feel, or that there really is no such thing as black and white, but because if we're to feel, inhabit and become sattva – holistic harmony at every level – we must first embrace these multitudes.

HERE IS ALL THAT MATTERS

With clarity we can begin to rethink the idea of *goals*. We've spoken of the way in which our lifestyles can follow our consciousness, and this is what we mean. We're all familiar with planning and goal-setting: 'In five years' time…'; 'After 10 years of hard work…'; 'If I put everything I have into this…'. The problem with goals is that our lives are, and have always been, *now*. We can talk of five or 10 years hence but they are at best projections and extrapolations and, when they do come around, we often find they've been complete fictions.

Dogged determination, single-mindedness and the very penning of a 'plan' assumes that we won't move from this path; so the fact that we've decided upon something can make us feel that we're locked into it, when in fact we may well reach a point where we shouldn't be hanging on in there. There is another way.

As our minds take on greater sattva and we grow our consciousness, we'll find ourselves more reliable. We'll trust our actions and decisions with less and less thought required and we will, more and more, be guided by our intuition. When we're balanced and well and able to strip away the unconscious blocks and samskaras – those old experiential scars – we'll simply see more clearly. As we do so we'll find the need for goals becomes more and more redundant.

This isn't about being unambitious or fostering a poor work ethic; although we may no longer find that hard work and the sacrificing of all our time correlate directly with success and productivity in the ways that we assumed. We might find that the amassing of wealth won't nourish our children as much as the time with them we might forfeit, or that following the expected path isn't the most meaningful route. All traditional routes are somebody else's story, after all; someone else's view of order.

When we live our lives in a state of openness and embrace the world as it comes, we'll find that we can *flow*. We'll better guide our selves and others and, crucially, we'll be better able to respond and adjust when obstacles present themselves in all areas of our life. This is the essence of Ayurveda – to prepare and endow our selves, to be responsive rather than reactive. In doing so we automatically prevent a great deal of what might damage us, we better serve others and we're able to blaze the most meaningful trails.

Have you ever experienced trepidation or anxiety before making a presentation or attending a meeting and believed that such feelings are somehow important and helpful – part of being 'prepared'? They aren't. We can perhaps avoid all mishaps by contemplating every possible eventuality or outcome and formulating plans for each. (We're exhausted even by the writing of it: mainly because we lived it for so long.) This is similar to the idea that we best support our immunity by killing off every external threat to it: mercilessly sanitizing every surface or perhaps avoiding stepping outside at all.

A much easier and more effective way is to bolster and support our foundation, the very basis of our lives – the terrain rather than the invader – and flow from the inside out.

Be Here Now

Our motion, a walk, can so often feel like simply a void between where we've been and where we're going. A walk can mirror our minds in this way. When our thoughts are of things that have passed and things to come, we are never *here*. Since neither the past nor the future exist – the one gone, the other not yet here – devoting our attention to that which is *actual* (spending time in the present) helps us simply to *be*. Incorporating this, and the discipline of *witnessing*, into simple actions such as walking can infuse a day with renewed clarity.

As we experience the present through our senses, we can feel it and intuit our way. It's neither a projection nor a memory. We can witness it and we can take part. A walk ceases to be limbo or a means between A and B, instead becoming a mindful experience of our journeying, connectivity, body, breath and surrounds. This is because our attention is with us rather than peripheral, disembodied or jumping forwards in time.

A WALKING MEDITATION

Like planting our bare feet on the soil, this practice is very grounding. It brings us back to Earth and into clearer awareness, and dispels residual anxiety and tension. Let's begin:

1. As you start to walk, concentrate on your breath. Breathe deeply and easily. Be aware of the number of strides you take to each inhalation. How many to each exhalation.

2. Spend a minute or two with this and feel the rhythm and connection between the strides and the breath. Try to lengthen each breath by one stride for each in-breath, and by one for each out-breath.

3. Be aware of what you can see, what you can hear; be aware of the feel of your feet on the surface of the ground. Be aware as a *witness*, without judgement or encouraging thoughts further than a recognition of what you see, hear and feel: birdsong, breeze, voices, rustle of leaves, sounds of traffic or machinery, blinking of lights. Be aware of your intuitive and bodily response to each. Allow it to be acknowledged; allow it to fade.

4. Be aware of sensations in your body – the synchronicity between your breath and your movement, the beating of your heart, heat or cold, any bodily aches and the thoughts that come. Again, be aware as a witness. Simply recognize the sensations and thoughts that come, and then return to awareness of your breathing. Neither direct nor suppress your thoughts. Only witness.

5. Stop for a minute or two. If the circumstances allow, remove your shoes and socks. Walk a short distance and then return. If there's a path and grass or earth, walk a little on the path, then back on the grass. Be aware of how this feels and the difference. Be aware of your surroundings, the sounds and sensations.

6. Close your eyes for a moment. Continue to breathe, deeply and easily. Lift your shoulders, to create space for the breath. Inflate your stomach as you breathe in. Empty it slowly and fully as you breathe out. Stand on the earth or the grass and, with each inhalation, understand that you're drawing in nourishment from the Earth through your soles, up through your body. With each exhalation you're expelling the stresses, anxieties and toxins that

have accumulated, through your body, through the soles of your feet, into the Earth.

7. Continue to walk in this way: witnessing your breath, your movement, the sensations, thoughts, sounds and surrounds. When you arrive at your destination, be aware of how you feel, of your body and of any changes.

HEART OVER HEAD

A simple reading of this maxim is that we should follow our intuition (heart) over our intellect (head) – be led by our emotional desires over a more analytical approach to path-finding. In the West, we prioritize goal-setting and planning – rational ways to get what we want – and devalue intuition and instinct: going with what 'feels' right. We 'set' our intentions in the same way that we might write our to-do lists – *thinking* about the things we want or need to work towards, and get. Ayurveda has a slightly different understanding of intention.

Intention is best defined as *sankalpa* – a Sanskrit word that refers more to a particular focus or positive promise than to a goal or plan; it emanates both from the heart and the mind and connects us with our highest truth. When we refer to the heart, Ayurveda understands this not as the beating organ that pumps our blood, but as the energy centre located in the middle of our chest – the heart chakra.

Intention, sankalpa, is powerful. It is potential energy, the seed of action and manifestation – carrying the full force of this action as a sunflower seed holds all the information pertaining to the flower in full growth and bloom. Ayurveda shows us that the mind lives in all parts of the body, and that intention is more powerfully initiated in the heart chakra, rather than in the over-thinking brain.

When we consciously apply focus and attention, our Prana (vital energy and life force) gathers around it – as in 'where attention goes, energy flows'. Prana can be channelled and directed. Intention is strengthened through the opening of our energetic channels, allowing Prana to flow ever more freely – clarity of intention and clarity of passage.

So where we place our attention, as in meditation or prayer, or when we focus on a particular aspect of healing, our energy gathers to support a clear intention. Equally, when our intentions are negative or destructive, these, too, are magnified by the gathering of our Prana around them. So clarity of intention is of great importance.

The use of ritual helps to open up our consciousness and the avenues for our energy, as well as to focus our attention without distraction. In Ayurveda, rituals such as the chanting of specific mantras during the harvesting, preparation and application of herbs, oils and poultices, are carried out to endow the preparations with vital energy and healing intention, and thereby magnify their efficacy.

Mantra helps in directing the healing energy of herbs into the human consciousness and the optimal energizing of the mind towards their reception. Without this 'spiritual' aspect, healing is only bodily and as such, limited and superficial. Under Ayurveda, however, healing is both a physical and a *conscious* act.

A RITUAL FOR SETTING CLEAR INTENTIONS

The practice of dedicated intention-setting is useful and, we find, a great beginning and end to a day. Let's begin:

1. Sit quietly and place your attention on your breath. Breathe deeply and easily.

2. Ground yourself by visualizing roots growing from the soles of your feet, anchoring you to the Earth, or by placing your bare feet on the earth or grass.

3. Bring your attention to your heart chakra: the area in the centre of your chest. Place your right palm here and your left palm on top of the right.

4. Allow a clear intention to form – a positive promise to yourself – and allow it to fill your heart. Avoid negative or harmful connotations to this. As in Wiccan tradition, suffixing your intention with 'harm to none' is helpful.

5. Sit with your intention for a minute or two.

Clarity of Intention

With practice, *life* can be a series of conscious acts where we harmonize our energies with that of the whole. Both sattva and tamas are inert. Like intention, they are potential energies that rely on the motion of rajas to be translated into action or effect. Sattva as a fundamental, universal force is understood as brahma or creative potential; tamas as *mahesha*: the potential for destruction. Through cultivating clarity of intention, we can follow the higher path of rajasic sattva (where we move towards greater awareness and purer states of consciousness) and leave those self-destructive behaviours and thought patterns behind us.

In many animistic and pagan traditions, ritual, sound, music, chanting and elemental forces such as fire or plant medicines are used to bridge the language barrier between humans and nature and to attain to more heightened and aligned levels of consciousness. This is often seen as, in a sense, a trick – inducing mind-altered states that impair our rationality. However, entering these states undoubtedly allows us to *feel* appreciably and profoundly connected to the whole and to directly experience new threads of perception.

Experiential clarity or heightened awareness – such as that gained through consistent Vedic, mantra-based meditation, or just simply *feeling* the importance or the truth of something as imparted – makes for difficult alchemy when we seek to fuse it with intellectual understanding. The efficiency with which we heal, or our levels of contentedness, compassion, anxiety and fear, however, are easier to measure, so take these as your best guide.

Again, feeling over knowing... clear as day.

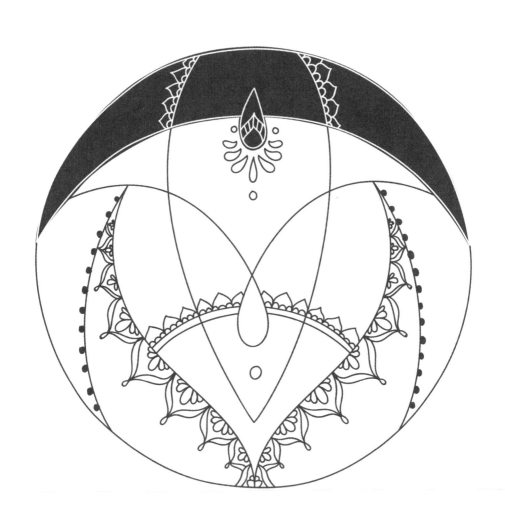

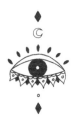

CHAPTER 6

GENTLENESS

'This earth is the honey of all beings, and all beings are the honey of this earth.'

BRIHADARANYAKA UPANISHAD

WHEN WE EMBRACE SATTVA, we come to think differently about our place in the world and, indeed, our impact upon it. A conscious choice from a good place, harmless and harmonious, is a truly powerful thing – such choices inspire community, create commonality and introduce wave upon wave of positive change. With our relentless rushing and juggling, busy-ness has become a truly modern malady: with plates overly full, we rely ever more on quick-fix convenience foods; the focus on surviving rather than thriving.

When stressed and rushed off our feet, we simply don't have the capacity to more deeply consider the alternative, or feel into the 'cause and effect' that is the true essence of karma. Yet, we know that every choice begets a consequence. In this chapter we pause to digest more deeply the energy and effects of sattvic food, and return to the roots of goodness and a true relationship with seasonal, unprocessed, whole foods – savoured and enjoyed, with gratitude.

NO PAIN, NO GAIN

There can be many shades of violence built into our lifestyles. There is, of course, true aggression, outright and knowing, but often, even for the placid among us who rarely aim to inflict harm, violence is more subtly woven into our cultures and our days. It can be made to feel virtuous and necessary, a fundamental component of successful living.

The simple Ayurvedic tenet of *ahimsa*, 'non-violence', becomes the most revolutionary of principles when applied to all these layers and shades. This is especially true when we understand that the object of our violence is most often our selves, and this affects the way in which we view and engage with the world on every level. By following the principle of consciously avoiding harm to our selves or others, we bring balance to all other principles. Remember – *So ham. I am that.*

Consider some of our bite-size maxims: 'no pain, no gain', 'dog eat dog', or the one with the omelette and the eggs. Each of these flies in the face of Ayurveda. Persistent platitudes such as 'no pain, no gain' can be extremely telling and badly need a little debunking. First of all, *pain*, as we know, is our natural response to damage. It tells us that the hot thing we're touching is causing harm to our hand. It cries, very clearly, *stop*! Our cultural resistance to this signal, however, can be seen in many commonplace aspects of our lifestyles.

When we notch up a mean session at the gym and push, press, sprint and snarl through the pain barrier, we tend not to believe that we've damaged ourselves. The body, though, tells us this in no uncertain terms. Lifting heavy weights builds muscle through tear and repair, and transcending the pain barrier is breaching limits that we should heed when we seek a balanced, sattvic lifestyle. While we feel briefly energized and adrenalized, ultimately we need to rest and recover; a process which, all too often, we don't allow ourselves in our aggressively regimented (and often self-inflicted) fitness programmes.

Similarly, when we work a 16-hour day, pull an all-nighter, cram for the exam or seek to blend the entirety of our day's nutrition into a smoothie and sink it on the way to the train station, Ayurveda understands that we're shocking our selves. The body, mind and spirit don't appreciate this kind of heavy-handedness, and we'll recognize their rejection of it more and more as we begin to take a conscious approach to our lifestyles.

Far from ushering ourselves along the route to greater wellbeing, we're landing a blow from which we need to recover.

The Power of Stillness

Regimens like these reflect that rajasic state of mind and culture, and the pain we feel is an indication of this. The explosive ways in which we tend to approach wellness reflect the fact that we feel compelled to keep moving.

We don't have time to be still or slow. We have an understanding that exercise, nutrition and the means to support our lifestyles are important. We've lacked the understanding, however, that each of these is best prefixed by the word *gentle*. Obsessively healthy is as oxymoronic as it sounds. Vaidyas (Ayurvedic doctors) often laugh when they suggest that exercise should be stopped at the point when perspiration begins, but it's only half in humour.

When our lives and minds are dominated by rajas we'll benefit greatly from finding moments for stillness and quiet, even, and especially, when our minds tend towards constant movement. We can clearly feel this imbalance when we stop our bodies but our minds continue to race, plan and worry – especially when we understand from a rational point of view that we would be better served by simply switching off.

When we're overstimulated and our minds overworked, stillness and quiet can feel extremely unsettling – a place where our deeper truths begin to reveal themselves. While we often seek to plug the gap by reaching for our phones or the remote control, this only shows the extent to which we need to cultivate and incorporate more stillness, silence and gentleness.

On the other hand, when our minds carry an excess of tamas, our bodies become increasingly divorced from our consciousness and our minds rest, not on the higher interplay between mind, body and spirit, but on the physical. A tamasic mind tends towards excessive body consciousness and excessive emphasis is placed on the importance of physical appearance: the building, shaping and sculpting of the body, as well as the amassing of material possessions – those tangible, measurable things of weight that are literal blocks in our path.

SATTVIC MOVEMENT

Ayurveda believes in exercise without damage, and kind, forgiving nourishment, which has everything to do with deep enjoyment and nothing whatsoever to do with guilt or punishment. We don't recommend anything that doesn't chime well with you, or must be swallowed down like medicine. Conscious exercise works with the mind and spirit. It opens energy channels and helps to harmonize, rather than amp up, the mind.

Gyms provide a cloistered, sanitized, climate-controlled environment for our active time – they set it apart from our lives in general, which are increasingly sedentary.

It's natural, however, for us to be spontaneously and incidentally active as we go about our day. As for our ancestors, exercise was a part of the whole; drawn equally from purpose and exuberance. Allowing ourselves to be physically purposeful and joyful is the best and most sattvic exercise for mind, body and spirit. A healthy body becomes a byproduct of a harmonious whole rather than a sole aim or a waging of war against the physical self.

For us this is found in spontaneously moving and stretching wherever our bodies take us – with a little more vigour when Kapha is heightened. We allow body and breath to lead us in greeting the day – moving easily through a few morning sun salutations. It's in growing a garden, digging and squatting or spontaneously dancing with our children; carrying them aloft. It's even in the sweeping of a floor or scrubbing of a tile, as much as it's in the taking of a sunset walk. When we feel joyful, or we feel a welling of energy, we might break into a little run or hop like a child or a rabbit, and when the opportunity arises we'll dive into the sea and take on the swell.

Neither of us is too grown up for a little tree climbing, and we find joy and magic in activities that flow from the body to the mind, like preparing food or chopping wood for the fire. We'll seek rooted, natural pursuits – a spot found to remove our shoes and take a quick barefoot walk or gently grounding asana.

When we feel tense or stressed, all the seemingly mundane, everyday activities can be infused with violence, whether we're applying it to the wood we chop, vacuuming furiously or attacking the spiders' webs in the corners. Stress and tension can flow both into and from aggression applied to everyday things. By consciously being in each task with awareness, we can recognize these outward signs of inner imbalance, and nurture lightness of hand and mind. Mundane tasks may then become pleasant rather than drudgery and their fruits won't take on the violence with which they were enacted.

See the Whole

The active sattvic is versed, intuitively, in moderation and balance. When we tune in, we understand that an excess of anything is something we must pull back from in order to restore balance. This is true of everything. We're often told of things that are extremely beneficial for us: whether it's exercise, kale, probiotic yoghurt or avocados. Each is only helpful when they haven't been used to excess and when they ring harmoniously with our dispositions and doshic balance.

Some may help on an individual, biological level while being damaging on a macrocosmic, global scale. For example, where the journey of an ingredient involves violence enacted upon landscapes, biodiversity, waterways or faraway workers. Taking a truly holistic view means acknowledging that this damage to the macrocosm isn't extricable from the microcosm. It is, in a sense, violence carried downriver. We expand on this later, when we talk about a modern view of sattvic food.

The guidance around contemporary 'wellness' can often be simplistic – given on the assumption that its receiver has only a small capacity for understanding. It can be sweeping – overgeneralized and homogenized according to the prevalent physical health problems of the populace, such as obesity or diabetes. We aren't seen as individual beings, either by authors or health ministers.

Guidance is also often over-commercialized. Health in all directions is a point of sale for millions of products, regimes, processed foodstuffs, books and magazines. To tell you that you don't need to, and actually shouldn't, buy their product, at least not in excess – or to be utterly transparent about ill-effects or contraindications – would run counter to its commercial impetus.

Crucially, most modern guidance suggests that physical, mental and spiritual wellness are largely separate areas and the remit of different professionals – just as we might have an eye, foot or back doctor.

Ayurveda doesn't recognize these divisions, but rather seeks to inform the conducting of the larger dance and the orchestral harmonizing of all aspects of our being.

Ayurveda understands that to characterize an activity or natural foodstuff as good or bad can be very misleading. While an avocado has various properties that are beneficial to human health, like most things it also carries a certain level of toxicity. Five hundred years ago, the Swiss physician and chemist Paracelsus said that 'All things are poisons, for there is nothing without poisonous qualities. It's only the dose that differentiates the poison from the remedy.'

Everything in Moderation

So while we take from the benefits, we must also allow ourselves to recover. The best way is to avoid eating anything all the time, however compelling its nutritional profile; to insist instead on variety and moderation and to learn to feel the effects on our holistic health more effectively.

Our hunter-gatherer ancestors eked out a diet composed of hundreds of different natural elements each week, each foraged in small amounts. Necessity and humility; a balanced place in a wider natural context provided the template for human dietary health. Nature provides, as we know. Many of us now have access to a whole wide world of food in both variety and quantity, but increasingly we've chosen only the latter. Modern Western humans usually take from this bounty in a much more limited way, immoderately consuming far fewer things.

When we decide that one ingredient is so good for us that we must eat it every day, we begin to run into problems. A morning round of #avotoast, for example, or a daily yoghurt both raise Kapha. Their heavy, moist properties eaten every day will lead to imbalance, particularly for people who are more Kapha in nature or vikriti, or when it's not balanced with food that's opposite, elementally and texturally.

We may become more lethargic and morose and tend towards excess sleep; our digestive fire may be dampened and thereby our immunity and mood, and we'll hold excess dampness and heaviness in our bodies. In the winter and early spring, when Kapha dominates environmentally, these effects will be magnified.

If our avocados aren't perfectly ripe, well-travelled or sprung from organic soils then toxins or ama will build up in our bodies too. Constant consumption of particular things doesn't allow us to deal effectively with their downside or excess. It's beneficial to have an understanding of the health-promoting properties of various fruits, vegetables, seeds, vitamins, minerals or antioxidants, but tuning into how we feel is much more important.

THE 20 QUALITIES

Under Ayurveda, all materials, actions, thoughts and intentions have clear qualities or attributes. There are 10 qualities and their opposites, making 20 basic qualities of all substance and action. These are closely linked to the three doshas and the three gunas, on which the basic quality will have an increasing or decreasing effect. Balancing these qualities in our daily lives – our food, our thoughts and our actions – is therefore a great aid to overall balance. Below is a list of the 10 qualities and their opposites:

◊ Heavy – Light

◊ Slow – Sharp

◊ Cold – Hot

◊ Oily – Dry

◊ Slimy – Rough

◊ Dense – Liquid

◊ Soft – Hard

◊ Inert – Mobile

◊ Subtle – Gross

◊ Cloudy – Clear

AYURVEDA: A BALANCED DIET

The nature of the 20 qualities lends itself extremely well to an intuitive approach to lifestyle. They are traits that we can easily recognize and already seek to balance. Think of a meal and its textures. If something is hard and dense, we often like to accompany it with something soft and wet in which to dip. We think to ourselves, *This dish could do with some crunch, or something zingy and sharp or light to offset the more stodgy nature of the whole.*

Pleasure and efficacy converge here – a meal of various, dancing, balanced elements is pure joy. While we might be told that, nutritionally speaking, a heavy curry or stew is best paired with brown rice, Ayurveda understands that lighter basmati rice makes for a better partner and a more balanced meal.

When we balance both the qualities of a meal and its tastes (rasas) – sweet, sour, salty, astringent, bitter and pungent – it helps us to maintain doshic balance through aspects that we're generally already equipped to recognize in our food. Since eight of these qualities relate to Vata, eight to Kapha and seven to Pitta (some of them increase more than one of the doshas), intuitively and thoughtfully weighing these aspects of our food will guide us well in maintaining overall balance.

As the 20 qualities relate not just to ingredients, but to all substance, thought and action, Ayurveda sees food in a wider context than simply that which fills our bowls. Food is everything that we take in: our inhalations, associations, impressions and excitations. Once they have entered our being, we set about assimilating and incorporating them and we reject what we cannot.

For thousands of years Ayurveda has emphasized the paramount importance of digestion. This extends to all aspects of our lives, but is particularly revolutionary when it comes to the food we eat, since the significance of this ancient wisdom has only recently begun to mesh with our modern understanding.

We're beginning to understand the profound symbiosis between the delicate bacterial balance in the gut and our immunity; and as such, the way our immunity can be eroded by the use of antibacterial sanitizers or the overprescribing of antibiotics. It speaks to the value of ahimsa that nurturing and cherishing the bacterial flora from which we're largely made, rather than warring with 99.9 per cent of bacteria, is best for our overall wellbeing. Too often we've chosen to fight the external invader rather than bolster our inner self, and this can extend to every aspect of our lifestyles.

Optimal Digestion

Our nourishment isn't determined by the nutritional profile of what we put in our mouths, but by what we're able to absorb and put to use.

We may be regaled with the most healing ambrosia from the heavens, but if it catches us unawares, or our digestive fire is dwindling, it will be largely leached from our being or settle undigested and become ama too. Simply put: good food isn't much use without good digestion.

The good news is that very simple changes can gently reinvigorate and rekindle our digestive fire, or agni. This begins, not with *what* we eat and drink, but *how*:

◊ Wake early.

◊ Drink a glass of warm water with a light spritz of lime or lemon or a coin of fresh ginger. If you're excessively Pitta, drink warm water only.

◊ Eat a warm, relatively light and easily digestible breakfast.

◊ Eat only when hungry.

◊ Avoid snacking between meals.

◊ Have your largest, most complex meal at lunchtime when digestive fire (agni) is optimal.

◊ Drink warm water throughout the day (at the very least at room temperature) and avoid iced drinks.

◊ Sip water when thirsty and during meals, rather than drinking large quantities before or after.

◊ Chew fennel seeds after meals or sip weak fennel or fresh mint tea.

◊ Eat your evening meal early, ideally around 6 p.m. and ideally three hours before sleeping.

◊ Eat fresh foods, freshly prepared and in season. Avoid excessive eating of leftovers (which are called *basa* in Ayurveda – dead food), as this heightens Kapha, and in turn, tamas, which brings on lethargy of body and spirit.

Eat in Context

Ayurveda generally holds that cooking food is preferable to eating it raw, since cooking unlocks the properties of ingredients to make them more available, more easily digestible and gentler in their delivery – requiring less of our energy.

That said, Ayurveda isn't fond of a generalization. It also recognizes the benefits of those fresh shoots of spring and summer, when eaten in as natural a state as possible. Wild or freshly picked organic leaves and herbs are great providers of Prana: our vital energy and life force. In the spring, various shoots appear that can be useful for a little natural detoxification and to shift the residual heaviness and excess Kapha of winter.

In warmer weather and with the rising Pitta of summer, our digestion is naturally quicker and hotter and, with the weather more temperate, we require less bulk nutrition. This can allow us to partake in those thirst-quenching salads, zinging with crunch and cool; however, we should do so moderately and according to an intuitive and educated understanding of our doshic balance at any given time.

Raw food raises Vata: those airy and ethereal elements of body and mind. Vata imbalance can be recognized in many ways: in literal, appreciable air – a certain gaseous quality to our digestive rumblings or a tendency towards that anxious flight of mind; in skittishness, dreaminess or broken sleep; in loss of weight or emaciation; in drier, duller skin and hair; drier, harder elimination or a brownish tinge to the tongue.

Ayurveda's Vedic sister Yoga places more emphasis on raw food in the dietary principles it sets out. This isn't disagreement but rather *context*. While they are inextricably entwined in many ways, Ayurveda, more than Yoga, is aimed at everyone, regardless of their current situation or state of bodily, mental or spiritual balance.

In a sense, and often traditionally, Ayurveda provides the platform on which a yogic lifestyle can be built. For most of us, at most of our starting points, our bodily balance must be addressed and our spiritual health will follow, or the two advance in tandem. Yoga, on the other hand, helps those who have chosen its path to move beyond the limitations of the physical body and body consciousness towards self-realization.

Fresh and wild food connects us to natural forces and helps us to access greater subtleties of mind through delivery of Prana and the increase in air and ether. Through long-term devotion to unified yogic practice we learn to control and direct the flow of Prana and gradually increase our digestive fire (agni).

In doing so we may not require so much nutrition in the traditional sense, since innate, cosmic energies are tapped into and channelled. Such a yogi may withstand conditions and imbalances that would ordinarily lead to ill health for those of us who live a '9 to 5' life. To reach such a level, however, requires a degree of asceticism and a very dedicated practice and lifestyle.

For most of us, even while we're seeking to strike a more spiritual path, attempting a jump to such a stage would be detrimental to our wellbeing. For ordinary folks and casual yogis raw food is best eaten moderately, kept to the warmest time of year and the middle of the day; and for us ordinary folk, the Ayurvedic diet is the best leg-up on our path to tangibly greater sattva.

Eat Consciously

Before taking even a bite of food, it's important to consider our relationship with it. Food is something to approach through the spirit as much as the mind and body. It's such a pleasure and a plethora. Natural ingredients, in their natural state, can connect us with the language of our natural world and our place in it. When we can involve ourselves in the whole process, from forest or field to fork, and plot to pot, we're actively participating in the whole process of digestion, assimilating into our being all aspects of a food's preparation and thereby better preparing ourselves.

Nature is full of playful clues, symbols and gestures. Walnuts look uncannily like the brain they are so effective in bolstering, while almonds are like eyes. If you squeeze a hypericum berry it bleeds to suggest its wound-healing properties. The explosive growth and poison of belladonna hints at the types of condition it's effective in treating.

There are many, many examples of this gesturing of nature towards its beneficence: cauliflower and broccoli for lungs; guava tree limbs evoking the intestines; a rosehip, the womb. The deep red of beetroot and hibiscus indicate their effectiveness for replenishment during menstruation. Silver birch trees move an incredible amount of water through their slender form, and accordingly, birch is an excellent remedy for water retention. The tree's youthful appearance and relatively short lifespan links it to rejuvenation, cleansing and to springtime.

Reconnecting with Our Food

When food comes in a plastic packet, trimmed, processed, shaped, cooked and ready, barring the pinging of a microwave, we gain time. We lose, however, our understanding of a meal and our connection with nature and its expression. As well as sacrificing much of its efficacy to shelf life, we're also caught unawares since, when we pick fresh herbs or pull roots, chop, sprinkle, spritz or stir our steaming pots, we're all the while preparing ourselves for a meal. We're salivating and producing digestive enzymes. We're exciting and readying the body and spirit so that when we sit to eat, we're both receptive and grateful.

Involving ourselves more, even in an incremental or gradual way – taking control of a few simple meals; growing a few herbs on the windowsill, or seeking out blackberries in the late summer or wild garlic in the spring, tasting a dandelion or two – will begin to invite our spirit into the eating and awaken our intuition. In doing so we entrust less of our food's journeying to faceless companies, use less packaging, ensure less waste and better digest the experience as a whole.

Seeking out organic and biodynamic produce where possible also deepens our connection with the land. Biodynamic growing was conceived by the Austrian spiritualist Rudolf Steiner in the 1920s as a response to depleted soils brought about by over-farming, the industrialization of agriculture and the widespread use of chemical fertilizers. It's a rich and holistic system that ensures deep connection and empathy with the land, the elements and the natural phases and cycles of the day, the moon, the seasons and the wider cosmos.

Biodynamic growing begins where the stipulations for organic growing end – it's organic growing that's painstakingly sustainable and deeply rooted in a wider understanding of natural forces. In this way it chimes very strongly with Ayurvedic principles, and this is reinforced by the way in which the biodynamic movement is once again gaining heartening momentum in certain parts of India.

At home, in the garden and at our village allotment, simple growing practices such as harvesting produce in the morning or planting seed in the approach to the full moon, using homegrown chamomile as a tea for the soil – to calm and support troubled plants – or fertilizing with nettles and weeds immersed for weeks in rainwater, help us to align ourselves with widely forgotten natural processes. It involves a certain reverence and thanks – integral to both Ayurveda and biodynamics – as growing, cooking and eating with love and gratitude increase our enjoyment and nourishment exponentially. They are the very best raw ingredients.

A SIMPLE MEALTIME MEDITATION

Consistently placing our awareness on the experience of a meal can bring profound change to the way we feel about food, and the benefits we gain from it. Making lunchtime into a conscious, mindful meditation can help us to digest in the widest sense.

1. Clear the area of screens and paperwork. Allow your meal to be all that is happening.

2. Sit to your meal and invite a little stillness – be silent for a moment.

3. Close your eyes briefly and silently express your thanks for this meal – made possible by nature.

4. Eat slowly, chew well. Consider each ingredient, each taste, each texture; the layers of your meal.

5. Consider each ingredient and the journey it's undertaken, from its source to your table.

6. On finishing your meal, continue to sit quietly for a minute or two. Consider how you feel and any changes.

Eat Responsibly

The growth in the amount that the average person consumes far exceeds the rate of population growth. Where the alarm bells sound most deafeningly is in the rate of population growth of the animals that are farmed for humans to eat.

Humans and the livestock we farm make up the overwhelming majority of the biomass of all mammals on Earth (96 per cent of all mammals are either human or farmed), with the biomass of poultry being about three times higher than that of all wild birds[16]. Only a tiniest iota of the planet is now left for those wild things that yet hope to live without human interference.

How we choose to eat is of enormous consequence in ways we don't always understand or anticipate. Emissions from livestock contribute hugely to climate change, great swathes of forest are cleared, ecosystems and ancestral lands are destroyed, biodiversity is increasingly threatened and plastic litters our oceans – all through the provision of our meals of choice.

Human population growth has an impact, but it isn't the overriding problem. More important are our choices: the extent to which we're conscious of the whole, the amount we consume and waste and the narrow range of specific things we consume at the expense of the variety enjoyed by our ancestors.

16   Bar-On, Y. M. et al., 2018. 'The biomass distribution on Earth'. www.pnas.org/content/115/25/6506

Then there is, perhaps, the most glaring moral and spiritual omission of our times. Monotheistic religions have historically sanctified our special, sacred status over all other aspects of nature (humanist as opposed to animist), whereas throughout its history, Vedic philosophy and understanding has rejected any sense that we're above nature.

Meanwhile we collectively overlook the pain and fear endured by the animals we industrially farm, as well as their subjective and emotional needs – such as the need for movement and to nurture their young: the very, most desperate, needs we humans feel. Nevertheless, we feel justified in ignoring these needs, perceiving animals purely as 'livestock' and administering to the physical needs of animals we mean to eat or milk only where it's necessary for productivity. Collectively, we're partaking in this cruelty to a greater extent year on year, widely choosing the cheapest options where this correlates directly with the poorest treatment and quality.

Sattvic Food: Nourish the Whole

A proper understanding of sattvic food involves all of these aspects, and is steeped in gentleness. While there are traditional sattvic ingredients, which we'll explore, fundamentally, a sattvic diet is conscious, vegetarian, seasonal and organic or wild.

The sattvic diet is nourishing, essential, fresh and sustainable, mild in effect and balanced in terms of the qualities of the ingredients from which it's made and the effect on the doshas. It emphasizes foods that don't overstimulate (rajasic) or slow us down (tamasic). Often referred to as 'pure' food, sattvic cooking is thoughtful, and prepared with love and care.

Ayurveda is forgiving and understanding. It will advise on the optimal use and quality of all ingredients and on how best to combine and prepare them, even if it doesn't recommend their use. Meat, fish and alcohol, for example, are never recommended for a healthy person. Occasionally, however, chicken broth may be recommended medicinally, as might herbal wines, where alcohol in very small doses acts as a vehicle to carry medicinal herbs quickly into the bloodstream. Ayurveda isn't looking to take away your bacon butty, glass of wine or morning coffee, but to provide you with advice that takes into account the *whole*.

While Ayurveda emphasizes dairy products such as milk and ghee amongst traditional sattvic foods, this has, at times, been misrepresented or at least abridged, since the provisos that accompany these make for very different products than the milk and ghee we find in our supermarkets.

For milk to be considered sattvic, the cow producing it must be treated with love and care. It must have good, spacious, organic pasture free of pesticides or chemical fertilizers, and milk may not be taken when the cow is pregnant. The cow is allowed to bond with its young and its calf must be allowed to suckle amply before surplus milk is taken. Ayurveda recommends fresh, raw, unpasteurized, unhomogenized milk, still warm from the cow and produced in accordance with ahimsa (non-violence).

If milk isn't freshly consumed, it should be refrigerated raw then boiled and drunk warm within a week or so. Under a traditional application of Ayurveda, therefore, milk produced under the conditions prevalent in our modern industrial dairies – with the use of pesticides, unnatural feed, genetic modification, antibiotics, poor treatment or separation of young, pasteurization or homogenization – cannot be seen as sattvic.

Under Ayurveda, milk is only recommended when it meets these gentle criteria – the health and happiness of the animal directly relating to the health and goodness of her milk. Veganism is not at odds with Ayurveda, and we can of course thrive without dairy. It is, where sattva is concerned, far preferable to consuming industrially produced milk.

A STEP IN THE DIRECTION OF SATTVA

And yes, we know, we know: this may all sound so far from so many of our social norms when it comes to modern Western food and lifestyle as to be impossible to incorporate. As we've said, everything is balance and the current balance is hugely off. Pure sattva – with complete absence of rajas and tamas – is completely unattainable and, in the context of a busy modern life, not desirable if we wish to be productive. But, the truth is, many of us swing without interruption from rajas (doing, racing, competing) to tamas (dulled-out, tired, passed out, weighed down, lethargic), with ne'er a moment of sattva in between.

We know, at first hand (and in our heart of hearts), how desperately this gentle, harmonizing, balancing energy is needed. Even if it's just a little, a baby step, bit by bit. For those reading this book, our recommendation is that you seek to consider and incorporate any small aspect of this guidance that appeals to you, and to adopt, not the whole practice, but the *direction*.

This is the essence of conscious choice – focused on intention over outcome. Incrementally, you'll find as we both have, that just one step in the right direction will naturally grow your holistic health, your consciousness and your connection with nature (especially your own) – and the next step towards greater sattva will feel innate and timely.

This may be in seeking out your nearest biodynamic farm, cutting out meat from one or two meals a week, or dabbling with vegetarianism. You may be drawn towards growing herbs on your windowsill or pressing some seeds into the soil to see what grows. It may be creating space to prepare a family meal lovingly, and to eat with thanks and reverence. It may be simply lending your thought and attention to the sections in this chapter; or sincerely reflecting on your societal or cultural conditioning – cultivating a little *satyagraha* – holding firmly to truth as it finds you.

It may be checking an ingredients list for certified sustainable palm oil, looking for a fair-trade emblem or buying a foraging book and taking a basket to the woods for a little gathering. Because, in these modern times, there's nothing that will do more to restore our holistic health and that of our planet than bringing greater sattva to the way in which we eat and consume.

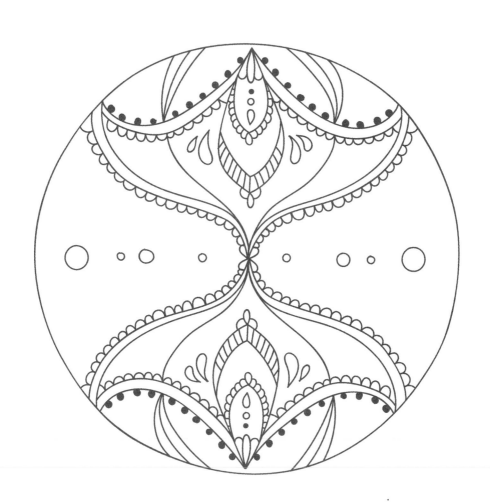

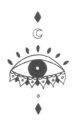

CHAPTER 7

SERENITY

'Earth's crammed with heaven,
And every common bush afire with God,
But only he who sees takes off his shoes.'

ELIZABETH BARRETT BROWNING

SLEEP CAN BE THE SILKEN WALL between entering the world with positivity and our days feeling darkened and difficult. It has transformative power over our waking lives. Here we withdraw into more subtle layers of consciousness where we're gently renewed. Sleep, or *nidra*, is a process and an order – one of the very pillars of Ayurvedic healing.

TO SLEEP, PERCHANCE TO DREAM

True, deep, replenishing sleep has little to do with falling into bed exhausted and everything to do with the preparative power of our lifestyles. The electric light and snooze button have shifted our experience from that of our ancestors who, after a good day's hunting, gathering, preparing, eating, playing, creating and communing, were guided into sleep by the setting sun, the hypnotic dancing of flames and the serene winking of stars. The stimulation that they had accumulated through the day – on their busiest days, so much less than we absorb today – was easily dispersed, and they settled down to sleep according to their needs and the natural light of the season.

Now we have a lot more to release. Our days are so often full of blue light, peripheral noise and endless entertainment – all those sticky jingles, bodily and chemical stresses and tensions, niggling worries. In the evening we have less of the slow, lulling, harmonizing motion of nature – less fresh air, more stimulants in our systems, more artificial light and modes of distraction that block us from uncoiling and unwinding. Our tiredness isn't joined by the preparation or background necessary for the sweetest ZZZs.

As we write, we're not afraid of the smartphone or the computer screen. We don't have it in for technology, social media or the electric light bulb, but we *are* aware of the need for balance and are fond of restful sleep.

The quality, layering and timing of sleep is of the utmost importance. There will be mornings when we wake, alive and exuberant after six hours, and days when a solid eight just doesn't feel enough.

A Sattvic Night's Sleep

Ayurveda has many natural, sattvic solutions to awaken your inner-morning person: to restore true serenity to sleep and bring back the dappled magic of a new morning. The following are just a few:

◊ Eating your evening meal early and fully digesting before sleep makes for a natural parcelling up of your energies. Ideally we should sleep at least three hours after eating, and dinner should be taken earlier and kept lighter as our digestive fire, agni, starts to slow after 3 p.m. Sleep is, in itself, *digestion*, as we assimilate the day's happenings and the incorporation of our physical food takes energy from that of our environmental nourishment.

◊ Being aware of your natural tendencies, dosha (prakriti), and any imbalances (vikriti) is extremely helpful for serenity of sleep. Kapha imbalance will find us tending towards too much sleep, feeling that leaden impossibility of hauling ourselves out of bed when the morning arrives.

Think of those dark mornings in winter and early spring when the season's humour is predominantly Kapha. This weight swells around the full moon and is best remedied by less sleep and earlier rising. Heightened Vata will make for disturbed, anxious sleep and that flighty, worried mind in the wee hours, especially in the late summer and early autumn. An excess of Pitta will bring sleep that's excessively hot and quick. We'll feel revived after only moderate sleep but depleted again later in the day. Balancing our doshas and disposition with our lifestyles generally will help to harmonize our sleeping patterns.

◊ When feeling Pitta imbalance, we should sleep on our right side; for Vata and Kapha imbalance, our left side.

◊ Where possible we should allow ourselves to wake naturally. This isn't such a pipe dream as it sounds, especially if we work on getting to bed early. Try setting your intention like an alarm – 'I will wake up at 6 a.m.' – ahead of your electronic one if you like. You'll be surprised how well this works. Leaving the blinds a little open and allowing a little ventilation will also help with this. Small signals, like a shaft of natural, encroaching light or the beginnings of birdsong, will help to bring us slowly and less heavy-handedly into the day.

DAYDREAMING

The feeling of waking serenity can be hard to come by in our modern lives, and particularly in our frenetic cities of pulse and buzz where the birds have lifted the pitch of their song in order to compete with the volume. In many ways this serenity is the culmination – the pinnacle – of Ayurvedic practice and of Yoga, and all of our sattvic steps are drawing us closer to it.

When we think of all the day-to-day aspects of our lives that are a barrier to peace, it can seem impossible that we'll achieve it in a lasting way. If we tilt our angle a little, however, we can see that it's our natural state: the point at which our lives and lifestyles begin, and ultimately where these lives will end. It's the impervious sleep of a newborn baby. It's our immediate destination when these bodies of ours are done.

In between we have a roiling sea of thoughts, desires, visions and noise that shift us from serenity. We have a build-up of trauma and events, impressions and associations that are constantly triggered, and we have projections, expectations, aspirations and plans to put to fruition before we can settle into peace.

The day brings many actions, reactions and interactions before we sink into our chairs in the evening and breathe, 'peace at last'; again, as the light and sound from the TV, the dull drone from the road, the flashes of colour through the gap in the curtains and the stream of alerts from our smartphones add to the huge overstimulation we've already received – many thousand times more than our hunter-gatherer ancestors.

And when we find that spot – a deserted clearing in the woods or the endless horizon devoid of electric light – and settle by the campfire, our minds are needled by the deficit (that hole in the ceaseless entertainment) and we become fearful and edgy, faced suddenly with deafening silence and with our true selves. Our thoughts race and we rummage in our kit for a phone to clot the hole.

It's become a bit of a cliché to say that true serenity can only be found within. We're not advocating withdrawal from the material world or worldly pleasure, but the cultivating of a spiritual state by which we can truly take pleasure in all our simplest worldly miracles. There are few places on this Earth of ours where we can be free of all man-made noise and reach, whether it's a distant aeroplane flying over the primary rainforest, a plastic bottle washing up on the most remote Patagonian islet or a telephone signal creeping into the desert.

Travelling to these places can be a very beautiful thing. The direct experience of nature's true, subtle, slow and expansive rta and resonance is healing and powerful, and we feel very privileged to have experienced a few such fragile, luxuriously natural places. Practically speaking, though, we can't always up sticks from our lives, nor do we leave our states of mind behind when we do. To truly live well, the serenity of sattva must be a layer of our everyday; part of the fabric of our lifestyles.

SANSKRIT: PURE EXPRESSION

We've used that beautiful, onomatopoeic word rta – the beat to which everything dances, order and rhythm. As writers we understand the importance of sound and rhythm, meter and cadence. The transporting effect of a thoughtful image, the lilting nuance of music or poetry that plays on our senses and physiology.

Sanskrit, the language of the Vedic civilization, is, in translation at least, the perfection of sound – complete, purified and sanctified. This is the original language of the Vedas, of Ayurveda and Yoga, which bonds the philosophies of Hindus, Buddhists and Jains and has infused so many of the tongues of Asia, not to mention our own. It touches our learning and our urban *jaṅgala*. It's the *jamiti* in our geometry, the *mātr* to whom we're born, the *śarkarā* – the very sugar in our bowl.

The sheer scope, economy and subtlety of Sanskrit slackens the boundaries of poetry and expression. When we try to describe a feeling, a spark of realization, a dream or the kernel of spiritual awakening, we can do so only in the language available to us. This is why we emphasize the importance of following *feeling*. There are many subtle things that don't lie within our language base or cannot be amply explained.

Sanskrit widened this panorama of expression so that it could be more broadly, more accurately and more succinctly rendered. This, as well as the numerical system devised in the Vedic era to accompany Sanskrit, aligns it remarkably well with the kind of algorithmic calculation used in modern computer science.

Good Vibrations

The power of words doesn't stop there. The pen is mightier than the sword, but the true paragon of language is sound – oral tradition, recitation, chant, music. Sound is not only meaning and expression, like words on a page. It also relates directly to action. We might recognize this in small ways through an understanding of onomatopoeia. When we *crack* a *stick* or *feck* a *block* into the next field.

More and more we're understanding that sound or vibration is the creative force of the universe, from which substance and matter is derived. This understanding pervades modern physics as much as it does the Vedas or the Bible. We can visualize the way in which sound gives rise to shape when different frequencies of sound are applied to water or sand to produce beautiful and mystifying geometries.

Where there is harmony and resonance of sound, there can be incredible healing; and equally, damage where there is dissonance. The frequency of the Earth's vibration for example – 7.83 Hertz or the 'Schumann Resonance' – brings great serenity and restoration. Time spent *grounding*, with our bare feet on the earth, and bathing in our natural surrounds helps to align our bodies and brainwaves with this pulse of the Earth, reducing their frequencies to those commonly generated during meditation or serene moments of relaxed mindfulness. This is the calming lilt of nature and its ability to slow and restore our minds. We are brought, literally, down to Earth. Grounding in this way produces a great feeling of safety and return.

Each element of our being has its own vibration. When in harmony, we're orchestral, capable of the most incredible creativity, beauty and reach. Where there is discord amongst our elements and our surroundings, there is blockage, a loss of cohesion within the whole and ultimately unhappiness and dis-ease. What is true of the microcosm, of course, is also true of the wider world.

VEDIC MEDITATION AND MANTRA

Sanskrit was born of serenity, received through meditation. The sound *Aum/Om* relates to universal consciousness, the primordial sound of the universe, and thereby the heights of human consciousness: the 'self' that is shared by all; the 'divine' from which all creation emanates and where we're all connected. It's from this strata of consciousness that the 'seed' or *bija* mantras used in Vedic, mantra-based meditation are taken.

Sanskrit syllables produce specific vibrations that relate to and stimulate different energy centres or chakras in the body; increasing energy, resistance and relaxation, flow of blood and related brain function. Different sounds play subtly and profoundly with different levels of consciousness, and place specific effects on the mind and nervous system of the reciter or receiver. Mantra is the legacy of this understanding.

If we look at the very well-known mantra Om Namah Shivaya, we can hear the effect of the mantra's syllables themselves – how they are inherently harmonizing and bring about a feeling of serenity. Not only are the sounds imbued with consciousness-raising resonance but their literal meanings are also illuminating. *Na* relates to the earth element, *ma* to water, *si* to fire, *va* to air and *ya* to ether. In this way the effect of the whole is one of balance and natural sequence – following the elements from the earth on up: that, ultimately, we are all one, in universal consciousness.

Om Namah Shivaya means 'salutations to the auspicious one' – a prayer offered up to the god Shiva. The use of gods or gurus helps in providing the right impetus and intention to access the energies of the sounds. This is the basis for the power of prayer. The gods are a part of an incredibly complex language – that of universal energy. Each represents an aspect of consciousness. Mantra, as Dr David Frawley explains, is 'energized prayer', where intention and sincerity are aligned with the natural forces contained in the sound.

One of our favourite mantras, and also one of the most ancient, is the Gayatri Mantra; this is approached as a devotion to *Savitur*, the divine power of the emerging sun – a sincere plea for knowledge as to the way that's right and good. The effects of the sounds on the mind are cleansing and purifying. Through repetition, the direction and trajectory of the sound is realized. In personalized mantra meditation, with each repetition we move subtly towards bliss – ananda – the mind's natural direction and resting place. As with sattva, bliss isn't the goal but the direction, the progress into ever-deeper healing, rest, love, happiness and compassion.

Often people in the West prefer practices where the use of mantra has been removed – for example, from the performing of particular yogic asanas. It should be understood, though, that mantra accompanying practice isn't an unnecessary or impractical religious attachment, but a powerful and integral means by which the practice is energized and directed, upwards.

Ayurveda considers meditation to be the main means by which to heal the mind and to relieve our selves of buried neuroses, fears and associations. It also helps with many aspects of bodily healing by working on the psychological roots of disease and imbalance. Meditation can be prescribed at all times without worry, where herbs or medicines, for example, may have contraindications.

Meditation is always most effective when grounded in Ayurvedic lifestyle, through sattvic diet and our external food of nourishing sattvic impressions and associations. Ayurvedic lifestyle naturally supports and furthers meditation in its healing and harmonizing of body, mind and spirit.

Nadi Shodhana

In Sanskrit *nadi shodhana* means purification of the pathways or psychic channels – it helps to open our bodies to the flow of energy. It's a part of the extraordinary ancient Vedic technique of 'rounding', which employs posture, breath and meditation (as well as appropriate lifestyle and nutrition) to open consciousness and bring on deepest healing and rest. A rounding retreat overseen by a qualified and dedicated meditation teacher will not easily be forgotten!

PRANAYAMA FOR SERENITY
– ALTERNATE NOSTRIL BREATHING

Nadi shodhana brings serenity to both the mind and the nervous system. It harmonizes the two hemispheres of the brain, and our masculine and feminine energy, and is an excellent technique for anyone suffering regularly from insomnia, headaches or high blood pressure.

Performing *nadi shodhana* for three to five minutes prior to meditating will noticeably deepen your practice and bring deep calm. Let's begin:

1. Before practising, make sure that your nostrils aren't blocked and your airways are free and easy. Sit comfortably and upright, and allow yourself a moment to become aware of your breath. Form a gentle fist with your right hand. Then extend your thumb, ring and little finger. This is *nasika mudra*.

2. Block your right nostril with your thumb and exhale slowly through the left nostril.

3. Keeping your right nostril blocked, inhale slowly through the left nostril.

4. Remove your thumb, block the left nostril with your ring finger and exhale through the right nostril.

5. Inhale through the right nostril, block the right nostril with your thumb and exhale through the left.

6. Continue to repeat these steps and end by exhaling deeply through the left nostril.

Repeat the process for a few mindful minutes, maintaining awareness of your breath. Try to slow and extend your breath a little as you practise, with your exhalation twice as long as your inhalation.

❧❧❧

The Doors of Perception

Higher, deeper consciousness is where we all meet: the source of life and intelligence. We're aware of our more superficial means of realizing our commonality, through the physical and emotional levels of consciousness – we can appreciate the sensitivities we've accumulated and our emotional reaction to somebody else's experience of the traumas and elations we've stored: what we call *empathy*.

We also have an understanding of the invisible and energetic ways in which we connect with and impact one another – how one person's mild panic or ill temper can quickly spread through a bus or train carriage on a cloud of pheromones and energy, or how something in a person's demeanour or presence can fill us with hope or dread. What we might call good or bad vibes. At the most subtle of physical levels, every interaction and observation is an exchange of particles; a fundamental and actual alteration that we effect or absorb.

We all exist within our ambits of perception. We have a visual ambit – those things of appreciable size and hue that our eyes allow us to see at particular distances. We have a scale of sounds available to our ears and a range of things that might land on our skin, which we have the capacity to feel before they flit or fly. Aside from the tastes that our tongues can discern, there are others that we cannot, but which are available to other species. Dogs will respond to whistles that play pure silence to us.

While some species see the world in black and white, others see it in much wilder technicolour than our own. Certain birds are thought to see magnetic fields, while bats and dolphins are masters of sonic impulse. Alarms (rather alarmingly) have been developed to prevent groups of youths from gathering – these emit noise that's painful for the young yet simply manifests as silence for older people, whose gathering and communing is presumably less distasteful! A fireworks display in broad daylight isn't materially different to the bonfire night spectacles to which we're accustomed, but the experience is completely different.

Experiential Consciousness

What is eminently clear is that there are limits to our sensory perception, and a great deal going on under our noses that goes unrecognized when we rely solely on these physical tools. This also raises a problem in describing the world and its phenomena in definite terms, since a colour, scent or even level of solidity may be different according to the being doing the perceiving.

Physics and mathematics can, rather beautifully, predict and describe aspects and energies of the universe that we're not able to view directly. At the most fundamental, quantum level, to 'observe' the most elemental particles is to interfere with them. We can, however, begin to grow our experiential consciousness. When we have the peripheral volume turned up high, as in our cities and satellites where the man-made sounds are incisive and the lights are bright, we've no eye or ear for subtlety. It's when we strip our world back and better manage our perceptual scapes that we begin to discern more.

As we allow ourselves to enter and occupy those higher, finer, more subtle states of being, as defined by Ayurveda's koshas, or layers of being (see page 150), we find ever more subtle and finer ways to connect; ever greater awareness, compassion and understanding, and ever more serenity that we will carry to others. Through meditation we enter the macrocosm and are able to directly appreciate the *whole*.

Through Vedic meditation, we begin to experience energies directly, both within and without, that our senses alone aren't privy to. Through time spent simply being, rather than doing, we open up our realms of experience. By being more subtle ourselves, we may appreciate greater subtlety. We feel and align ourselves with natural rhythms previously obliterated by the freneticism of our days, the bleating of our tech and the hollers from the advertising hoardings.

MOVE TOWARDS ACCEPTANCE

Serenity, if we're to achieve it, is rooted in acceptance – acceptance of and gratitude for what we already have. We can spend a great deal of time focusing on negative things that come along, considering the shape of their negativity and the potential for further negativity. Imagine if we devoted the same amount of time to appreciation of the positive things; if we allowed good things to expand and fill up the space that's currently occupied with the negative stuff.

In looking to achieve miraculous things and to ascribe meaning to our lives we can easily forget the miracles we witness every day and the great beauty of the world that spins before our eyes; the many blessings that we not only fail to count, but also decide don't count because we're busy pursuing others. It's in accepting and embracing our lives as they are, in truly occupying our blessings, that we give the world meaning.

Sunshine has no meaning until we feel it on our skin or receive its energy through our eyes. The seasons have no meaning if we've no time to savour their subtle turning and timely beneficence. Our lives have no meaning when we're not present in them: grateful, mindful and accepting.

As Dr Vinod Verma, an Ayurvedic doctor and author, has so wisely explained, 'The first priority of Ayurveda is life itself.' First comes our entry into the world, our bodily and spiritual health, a peaceful, sattvic state of mind and a harmonious relationship with the world around us. It's *after* this that we move to the next priority of seeking means by which to sustain this life.

This is the opposite of the belief that we should first seek success, financial security, a well-paid job and assured growth, and then we'll be well placed to begin to live. By prioritizing life ahead of the means by which it's supported, we find that our lifestyles, our work and our ambitions are full of meaning because they are rooted in our life's essence and purpose. Our life and lifestyles are aligned.

When we're rushing, racing, reacting and competing with others for success, we're entirely overwhelmed by rajas. We're propelled by wind and fire, aggression, competition, and have no understanding of our own dharma – our higher purpose and soul-aligned work. We operate entirely on the terms of others and have no life of our own from which to begin. When we work, single-mindedly, to own things, achieve material wealth, purchase new clothes, shoes, cars, and assess our 'value' in this way, we're very much weighed down by tamas. We're heavy with 'stuff', ownership, clutter, trophies.

Sattva, then, is self-care at its most pure and conscious and connected. It's the stillness and serenity in which we find ourselves. It's not the single act of replenishment to offset a truly terrible and challenging day – it's the mindset that transforms the truly terrible day into one that we learn from and are far less affected by.

It's not a quality we allow into the beginning of the day and the end, the weekends and bank holidays. It's both the means and the end. It's the still, quiet centre of our entire lives that creates and illuminates the whole. It's the consciousness that puts the magic back into the plainest moments and makes the struggle evaporate.

SERENITY WITHOUT EXPECTATION

We're both as pragmatic as we are intuitive, and we know that, even with our best intentions, life doesn't always go to plan. Sometimes we'll wake up with a big smile, full hearts and lovely ideas – and our children will wake up grumpy, tetchy and impatient. Weekend after weekend passed by with a similar pattern repeating itself, and it really challenged our family's patience and happiness.

Why, we wondered, when we work so hard to create an environment of ease and light, did our children wake up in a bad mood? It wasn't until we meditated on things for some time that we realized we were very strongly imposing our expectations on our children – and that doing so brought stress, pressure and worry into our lives. We can no more engineer a perfect sunset than we can another's sunny mood. But we can – *you* can – decide to set intentions for your self in a way that's entirely removed from your expectations of others.

This is a very important facet of sattva – because it comes from you, from your heart and your essence, and is wholly removed from your ego. Intentions are most powerful when unconditional: when we simply want to live in a conscious way because it's the right and natural thing to do, not because we believe it will deliver us a specific end goal or reward (e.g. love, beauty, wealth). Expectations, on the other hand, are inherently conditional. We imagine what we want to achieve or receive from life, based on what we need, want or lack.

Sattva can be found in people who are accepting, not needing. Equanimous rather than expectant. It can be helpful to feel into your heart, and ask yourself:

◊ 'Is this my best unconditional and loving intention for myself?'

◊ 'Or is it my conditional wish, based upon what I expect to receive in return?'

Remove your intentions from your expectations, and you very naturally begin to separate your essence from your ego. Your essence will bring you greater sattva; your ego will not.

SOWING THE SATTVIC SEED

When we begin with *life itself*, we open up a natural path of 'spiritual growth' where our lifestyles shoot from that sattvic seed, embedded in our holistic health, personal truth and happiness. Meaning is built into the very foundations of life, and life is a process of nurturing and refining the plant as it grows. When we begin, however, with *the means* – with financial security and homogenous modes of success and attainment – we find this spiritual growth replaced by a path of actual growth or expansion that closely mirrors the dominant humanist and economic systems of modernity.

We assume that there's something at the end of this growth, or a point at which it's fully grown. There isn't. It's the only meaning attached to our lives – more money, more renown, more property: more power. Our income allows us to buy a home, but we must have a second – we must work harder and earn more to pay for it, but ultimately it will grow our money and the extent to which we're appreciably 'successful'. If growth is success then stillness is seen as stagnation – which is simply not true.

We have a friend we both adore who told us that she had no desire to grow her homemade business. It supported her and her family, was enjoyable and sustainable, and she could control the quality of her products. Her work was aligned with activities that she found pleasurable and fulfilling and allowed her time to spend enjoying her family, playing with her children and unwinding in the evening.

It sounds pretty perfect, a great blessing. But the fact remains that, when she says she doesn't wish to grow her business, most business people look at her as if she's lost her mind. Growth is the only creed that makes any sense in modern economics. Without assured growth, the whole system would collapse tomorrow. To remain still is failure.

This is how many of us are living. Our only understanding of success is to accumulate, to fill our houses with possessions, because these are the only way to gauge our value. We can pay for them incrementally on a long timeline and they will live in every room of the house, quietly detrimental and heavy.

When we 'outgrow' that house, we'll buy a larger one. As we do so we'll work harder, longer and under greater pressure to meet all the accompanying demands. Our holistic health will suffer and we'll deny ourselves even the most fundamental supports of life. We will forgo nourishing food and time to eat and digest. We will forgo fresh air for the conditioned kind that cycles around our offices. We will forgo meaningful community. We will forgo proper rest and sleep.

The only essentials in our lives are already abundant – water, food and air; and the best stuff is also free: love, nature and community. Our lives and myths have been making our primary needs secondary; solutions to be sold back to us. There's great liberty to be found in the simplifying of this equation. Like so many aspects of sattva, it's the taking back of those natural provisions that are our birthright.

Defining Spirituality

Throughout this book we've spoken a lot about the spirit, spirituality and spiritual practice. This isn't an invocation of the supernatural, nor is it theistic. Organized religion is prescriptive, by virtue of being organized – requiring submission to a particular doctrine and a certain amount of blind faith: belief in that which cannot be directly experienced or seen.

Often a creator is conjured who punishes or rewards on very human terms. Theists often concentrate on the points at which scriptures diverge – a particular swing from the common root that sets a group apart, or seeks to validate their special status: the chosen people; the sole keepers of *truth*. Division over unity… the self-aggrandizing work of the ego.

If you substitute the words 'creative force' or 'aspect of consciousness' for the word 'God', then the idea that a person might not believe in God starts to sound a bit strange. In India there are many traditions under the umbrella of Hinduism, and many gods, as there are many creative forces, many facets of consciousness, and many spirits of nature in animistic traditions.

In many ancient Indian traditions, for example, the god Shiva relates directly to Purusha, or purest consciousness, and the goddess Shakti to prakriti, energy or pure nature. They represent the most fundamental universal forces and the 'male' and 'female' qualities of all creation and are entirely equal and essential in their primordial magnificence. This is similar to the images of 'The God' and 'The Goddess' in Pagan traditions and the 'Old Religion' of Wicca and Druidism. As all creation is derived from the combining of these forces, all other gods and goddesses are aspects of Shiva and Shakti – of consciousness and creative energy – and formed of their interplay.

A big reason for this is to invite people to channel their devotion towards something that appeals to them individually. Often it may be another person – a respected teacher or family friend – rather than a 'god'. This is because devotion, or bhakti, is important – a voicing of our appreciation and love for life itself in all of its incredible multiplicity.

So, if you're less than delighted with the single image of a God – who is perhaps human-shaped and bearded, of patriarchal bent or rather vengeful and discriminatory – it may well be difficult to find motivation towards devotion. To be spiritual is to seek truth, and to understand that truth cannot simply be told but must be experienced. It's *satyagraha* – holding firmly to our truth as it presents itself. This word has often been interpreted as 'non-cooperation' when associated with Mahatma Gandhi, who coined the term, since the holding of our truth is often in direct conflict with prevailing myth.

We may believe that truth-seeking is the basis of science, and Ayurveda is science first and foremost. However, modern science seeks knowledge and innovation according to the prevailing concerns and priorities of the times, as well as commercial concerns and the matters most pressing to those most influential. It is commissioned and directed. Science depends on spirituality to define the scope of its enquiry and focus.

The spirituality that runs through Ayurveda ensures that its focus is holistic, that it's rooted in non-violence and that human health isn't separated from the health of the whole and the harmony of nature. It safeguards against unsustainable practice or methodology that advances modes of cruelty, complacency or hierarchy. It doesn't share the religious or humanistic view that human beings are meant to exist apart from and above all other beings.

Bow to the Truth in You

Recently, the adjective *post-truth* has entered the modern lexicon. There's a sense that literal truth has started to matter less and less. Truth, aside from natural law, has always been an energetic entity. Its veracity depends on the way in which it enters our consciousness.

A declaration might inspire our disagreement or our highest praise; capture our imagination or light the taper of our most vehement outrage. It depends on the level of consciousness at which it's received. As we invite greater sattva into our lives, we'll increasingly, steadily, attain to higher levels of consciousness. It's here that we'll find our truth, our ease, our serenity, our meaning and our flow.

We both believe in spirituality. We know that human beings are narrators, storytellers, and we know from the darkest of our days that living lives unduly propelled by rajas and disproportionately weighed by tamas muddies the tone of our stories. Ill health and imbalance on each of those bodily, mental and spiritual planes skews every piece of information we offer and receive. Sometimes we've held these positions for so long that it feels almost impossible to give them up or to accept that they have darkened and obscured the world we view. Sattva, then, is a spot of window cleaning. Polished glass, through which we can clearly see.

Through the gods of nature and consciousness, those *devas*, we see ways of relating to the world, to the qualities of the universe – and every aspect of our nature. We see channels for our devotion. To be grateful for, humbled by and devoted to the whole that we and every other being together comprise. In many of the beautiful teachings of ancient India, we see our best hope for humanity.

When we share that Namaste, with our palms joined at our hearts, we're expressing our recognition of the divine in one another – the understanding that 'I am that'. *So ham* – the natural sound of our breath – and so are you. Our devotion knows no hierarchy, no subjugation, no inequality or ownership. We are all 'that' and our devotion is towards the whole of creation, including our selves.

THE WHOLE STORY

'A human being is a part of the whole, called by us 'Universe',
a part limited in time and space. He experiences himself,
his thoughts and feelings as something separate from the
rest – a kind of optical delusion of his consciousness. The
striving to free oneself from this delusion is the one issue of
true religion. Not to nourish it but to try to overcome it is the
way to reach the attainable measure of peace of mind.'

ALBERT EINSTEIN[17]

---

17   Calaprice, A. *The New Quotable Einstein*; Princeton University Press, 2005, p. 206

Writing books about the *whole* is notoriously hard. It's so much easier to pitch a simple book into a simple nook, wherein it finds its pre-labelled spot on the shelf in the local bookshop. Cookery. Gardening. Diet. Exercise. It's been so very important to us both, though, to give ourselves up entirely to this idea that we've been carrying around in our minds and living within our lives for upwards of 10 years now.

Because there is no nook for this book. A nook-book will aid you in getting a tasty meal on the table, deepening your practice of Yoga, or advising on when to get your seeds into the soil, but it's not a blueprint for the whole you, or the whole of life. It's just a fragment… and we didn't want to write a fragment.

Instead, we really wanted to write a book that focused on *connecting* the pieces; to present a truly holistic way of living and being that joins all of the dots within and around us, and makes that process practical, enjoyable and beautiful. Possibly the most beautiful thing about Ayurveda is that it has never really limited itself to Ayurveda. It doesn't close itself to any aspect of healing.

Where Sanskrit seeks to perfect sound in the widest possible terms, Ayurveda seeks *complete* healing by opening itself to, simultaneously, the most subtle and the most expansive of healing landscapes: it connects and integrates. The sattvic lifestyle is *full* of possibility and you're invited to choose the aspects that appeal directly to you – to be seekers and spiritual expeditioners; storytellers. To find deepest serenity and connection, wildest magic and joy.

Finally, you're invited to do all those things that you may have done as children – to view the woodland from a treetop, to lie on your back in the long grass, to form pictures from clouds, to connect the stars, and to understand from these exchanges that such languages are as valid, as complex and as revelatory as any other, whether it's Sanskrit, algorithm, mathematic equation or the Queen's English.

A Return to Human Being

Much has been written on the distinction between the two parts of our selves: the essence and the ego. Our essence is our *spirit* – the simple, guiding, unthinking and shared force; our highest selves who are governed by intuition and tend towards unity. This is who we are at the very core of our being, and it's where all the lines and limitations begin to blur. It's where the physical body is transcended and we cease to rely on things that are solid and material. It's where our own interests, our health and happiness, converge with that of everyone and everything.

The ego is our busy minds, overly focused on how we're perceived, how we wish to be 'seen' and what we achieve. Almost all of us today are living in an uninterrupted ego state, or ahamkara. All that separates the two is awareness. An awakening to feeling. An opening of the heart to the goodness in your self, in others, and – though it may seem impossibly hard at times – in every situation too. A removal of our egoistic 'wants' from our simplest, spiritual 'needs'. The seismic but subtlest shift from doing, doing, doing to only *being*.

The aim of Vedic living is to enable us to perceive this 'higher reality'. But to get there, we first need to lay the foundations. A muddled, busy, anxious mind won't be ready to perceive anything beyond its own immediate situation. So, we need to clear the path, and the mind, so that it's silent and receptive enough to perceive the 'truth' within our own lives.

If you've ever experienced a bout of wonderful decision-making, chances are it was at a time when you had taken the time to rest, reflect and *feel* into a situation – which led to a much clearer perspective (there's a reason that so many people go away on holiday, sit by the sea, sleep, rest, breathe, and then return home and quit their life-sapping jobs).

At times such as this, we may also get an almost immediate result that helps us to trust that we've made the right decision (for example, we finally quit the job that we've long dreaded and a dream project comes out of the blue, shortly after). And, if this might all begin to sound incredibly poetic but somewhat unattainable, we'd ask you to think about a time, any time, when *you* have already felt this.

Because we've all felt it at times – that clear, light, thankful, positive energy as we step back from the daily fray and really absorb the loveliness of a particular moment. When we get a sneaking suspicion that taps us on the shoulder, as if to say, 'when you smile, the whole world smiles with you'. When we begin to feel that life is actually on our side, or indeed, the universe has our back. We finally let our guard down. We stop fighting, fearing and fretting.

We move, seamlessly and painlessly, from day to day, our own best intentions at heart, and realize that this isn't selfish. Your best intentions are aligned with those of the world around you too. To be truly generous and accepting of yourself is also to be incredibly generous to others – it's a warm smile, an unconditional welcome, an embrace. All around you will feel it, and want to remain close to it. If things come from a good place, they are almost always received in the same spirit. When we say that love heals, this is what we really mean.

'When all the senses are stilled, when the mind is at rest, when the intellect wavers not – then, say the wise, is reached the highest state… he who attains it is freed from delusion.'
KATHA UPANISHAD

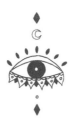

AFTERWORD:
WHERE OUR STORY ENDS
(AND REALLY BEGINS)

*'The meaning of life is just to be alive. It is so plain
and so obvious and so simple. And yet, everybody
rushes around in a great panic as if it were necessary
to achieve something beyond themselves.'*

ALAN WATTS

TODAY, AS WE GO ABOUT OUR LIVES – as we dig the earth, chit potatoes, grow and cook, tackle the tasks and the school run; sleep, eat and play, warm ourselves by the fire, laugh and dance – we're more and more led by a new mantra, the radical and simple words: 'I do not want anything more than I already have.'

Like everybody else we'll become sad, imbalanced, de-energized, and be confronted with difficulties, loss and unforeseen trauma. Our comfort is that we'll feel all these things and know that they will pass like the weather; that we have tools that allow us to adjust, balance and heal. When we don't know what to do, we'll do nothing – extend the space between stimulus and response.

When we look upon these life cycles of ours as those of disconnected individuals, they don't make sense. Of life we have said a great deal... but what of death? The searing pain of inexplicable loss and the weight of grief, held in the stomach and heart, unshifting, black as coal; the wrench of a loved one, taken from our arms – no words ever quite right as we fumble and curse and howl at the gods.

We've been there. We've lost dearest loves and there are still rivers of tears to be cried that we doubt will ever fully recede. How we miss the loves we so cherished. How we wish they would return to us. This is nothing but human.

> 'When you feel the suffering of every living thing
> in your own heart, that is consciousness.'
>
> BHAGAVAD GITA

We are made to love and ill-made for loss, it seems. Death can seem cruel, unfair, governed by bias or devoid of meaning. But... when we look at the whole, a bigger picture starts to emerge: the sharing and scattering, demise and distribution that allows for the continuation of life and the timeless unfolding of creation.

Creation and dissolution are aspects of the same expression. Ancient Himalayan Tantric and shamanic traditions teach that, as we approach death and our bodies become frail, senses weaken and thoughts are quieted, the essential underlying consciousness developed during our lives is uncovered and realized. While some are tormented by the cacophony of spectres it contains, heightened consciousness brings peace, acceptance and understanding.

If we see our selves as ONE – all of us, ONE energy, one consciousness, one being – we begin to perceive something of our true nature.

Our simple hopes lie in seeking to flow with this unfolding – gratefully playing amongst the many wonders of nature and finding the magic in all the small, simple stuff of the everyday. Being present and joyful in these things and these lives that are happening at every moment: the symphonic clatter of rainfall, a giggle that won't be stifled, the aromatic breath of rosemary, the softness of another's fingers, knitted through our own.

'Until we realize the unity of life, we live in fear.'
THE UPANISHADS

We will savour the beauty in both the miraculous and the mundane and all those spaces in between, sparkling with infinite possibility. There is no sattva at the end of this proposed path – no 10 steps to take us there –

only the path through life itself, which offers us two choices: consciously choose to move closer to the light, the goodness, the kind and the gentle, or choose to ignore, fear or diminish it.

A rose in full bloom today will begin to wither and die tomorrow. It will follow this cycle every time – from root and stem to bud and bloom – without question, without fear. It blooms no less exuberantly on the final day of its fullness than it does on the first – it blooms because it's made to bloom, just as it fades and falls because it's made to die. It is what it is.

What if the rose believed that there was no point – why put all of its energy into unfurling its promise-filled bud only to have its precious petals trodden underfoot weeks later? Then fear would win – and we would have a world without flowers.

The beauty and pleasure and truest meaning of sattva – purest consciousness – comes not from our focus on where it's taking us and what we'll do once we get there. No – purest SATTVA comes, simply, from trusting our selves enough to be who we always were, and to let everything else go.

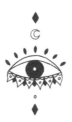

SATTVIC RESOURCES

Here you will find some background information on the sources we've studied, learned from and shared, and those wonderful Ayurvedic and holistic resources that we hold dear and refer back to often.

WHAT ARE THE VEDAS?

The Vedas are believed to be the oldest writings in the world. The word *Veda* means knowledge in Sanskrit – the ancient language in which the Vedas are written. The Vedas hold the beginnings of Indian philosophical, spiritual and medical traditions.

Composed of expansive and illuminating hymns, the Vedas hold universal truth and wisdom as understood and recorded by the ancient rishis (seers and sages), who shared it via the oral tradition, mouth to mouth, from the onset of time to the point at which the Vedas were formally written down – mostly, it's believed, by one man, Vyasa Krishna Dwaipayana – around 1500BCE.

The Vedas are made up of four sacred texts that house the roots of all wisdom that brought us Ayurveda:

◊ The **Rig Veda**, the book of mantra – including hymns devoted to 33 different gods, mostly of nature, from Agni (god of fire) to Indra (god of rain).

◊ The **Sama Veda**, the book of chant – derived from the eighth and ninth books of the *Rig Veda*. Filled with mantras, this is an exacting and instructive text that's meant for use during religious ceremonies and rituals.

◊ The **Yajur Veda**, the book of ritual – once again, this was written to guide those who carried out ceremonial religious practices, such as chants to cleanse and bless the instruments used during the rituals.

◊ The **Atharva Veda**, the book of spell – this is known as the 'wisdom of the Atharvans' and is filled with incantations to help those achieve their dreams and desires.

Within each Veda is a section called **The Upanishads**, which houses the philosophies of the Vedas and provides a spiritual vision for humankind, underpinned by practical and philosophical guidance to help us transcend our bodily limits.

Yoga, which originated in the *Rig Veda*, wasn't focused on asana (Yoga postures and movement) but rather on mantra (sounds and words). These mantras were sung without interruption by the rishis in a bid to unite humanity with the highest powers of consciousness within the universe.

Ayurveda first came into being as a series of Vedic mantras – it was not a fully formed standalone science within the Vedic texts. Instead, it's an Upaveda, or supplemental text, that sits within the *Atharva Veda*, and it's filled with mantras that relate to healing and wellbeing. It's not, however, confined to the *Atharva Veda* – as Dr David Frawley points out, 'aspects of Ayurveda can be found in all the Vedas and are inherent in the Vedic deities (devatas)'.

RECOMMENDED READING

It's with deepest humbleness that we give sincerest thanks to our teachers. Dr David Frawley, from whose works we've quoted and learned so, so much, and to him for creating the rich, instructive and illuminating Vedic Healing course at the American Institute of Vedic Studies, which brought a whole new depth to our understanding of this most subtle and beautiful science. And the legendary Dr Vasant Lad, all of whose books we treasure, reread and refer to almost daily – for your wisdom, humility, generosity and truth. We highly recommend watching the documentary about Dr Lad too – *The Indian Doctor*.

Below is a list of all the books from which we've learned; we'll continue to update it at www.thisconsciouslife.co, as and when new titles come into our lives:

Ayurveda

A Pukka Life, Sebastian Pole

Absolute Beauty, Pratima Raichur

Ayurveda Lifestyle Wisdom, Acharya Shunya

Ayurveda: Ancient Wisdom for Modern Wellbeing, Geeta Vara

Ayurveda, Nature's Medicine, Dr David Frawley and Dr Subhash Ranade

Ayurveda: The Science of Self-Healing, Dr Vasant Lad

Ayurvedic Astrology, Dr David Frawley

Ayurvedic Healing, Dr David Frawley

The Book of Ayurveda, Judith H. Morrison

The Yoga of Herbs, Dr David Frawley and Dr Vasant Lad

Sanskrit Texts

The Bhagavad Gita

The Mahabharata

The Ramayana

The Rig Vega

The Upanishads

Holistic Wisdom and Wellbeing

Body Wise, Dr Rachel Carlton Abrams

Eastern Body, Western Mind, Anodea Judith

The Effortless Mind, Will Williams

Elegant Simplicity, Satish Kumar

The Five Side Effects of Kindness, David H. Hamilton

How Your Mind Can Heal Your Body, David H. Hamilton

Intelligent Yoga, Peter Blackaby

Limitless Sky, David Charles Manners

Live Well, Live Long, Peter Deadman

Whole Beauty, Shiva Rose

Yoga Mind, Body, Spirit, Donna Farhi

Women's Bodies and Cycles

Code Red, Lisa Lister

Love Your Lady Landscape, Lisa Lister

Moon Time, Lucy H. Pearce

Our Bodies, Ourselves, Boston Women's Health Book Collective

Period Power, Nadya Okamato

Wild Power, Alexandra Pope and Sjanie Hugo Wurlitzer

Womancode, Alisa Vitti

Women's Bodies, Women's Wisdom, Dr Christiane Northrup

Yoni Shakti, Uma Dinsmore Tuli

Ayurvedic Cooking

The Ayurvedic Cookbook, Amadea Morningstar

East by West, Jasmine Hemsley

Eat Feel Fresh, Sahara Rose

Eat Right for Your Body Type, Anjum Anand

Eat. Taste. Heal, Thomas Yarema

The Modern Ayurvedic Cookbook, Amrita Sondhi

Ojas, Nira Kehar

What to Eat for How You Feel, Divya Alter

USEFUL WEBSITES

www.thisconsciouslife.co – this is our Ayurveda and Conscious Living blog, where we share recipes, features on holistic wellbeing, rituals for the spirit (spi-rituals), soul-nourishment and creating a sacred home space.

www.banyanbotanicals.com – this Australian brand has a fantastic, content-rich website where there's lots to read and learn.

www.jasminehemsley.com – Jasmine's My-Urveda section features interviews with practitioners and personalities in the Ayurvedic and wellbeing worlds. The online shop is also a great holistic retail destination.

www.ayurvedapura.com – this UK-based school, run by Dr Deepa Apte, also has a wonderful online shop that sells excellent remedies including chywanaprash; it is also rich in learning resources.

www.vedanet.com – The American Institute of Vedic Studies, founded by Dr David Frawley, isn't only the home of their online learning resources, but is also rich with free content – simply click on Knowledge Center.

www.ayurveda.com – The Ayurvedic Institute, founded by Dr Vasant Lad, is rich in free resources, including features and videos, and wonderful for all those seeking a way into the science of life.

www.maulirituals.com – practical reads and resources sit alongside their beautiful all-natural and award-winning wellness and beauty range, created by Anita and Bittu Kaushal.

www.samayaayurveda.com – an award-winning, all-natural, dosha-specific skincare range created by Abida Halstenberg.

www.pukkaherbs.com – a global wellbeing brand specializing in fair-trade herbs and teas, co-founded by Sebastian Pole and Tim Westwell. Global shipping.

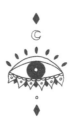

GIVING THANKS

From that very first day in March 2018 when our wonderful agent, Hattie at Blake Friedmann, called to tell us that our book had found a home at Hay House, we've become very intimately acquainted with what things feel like when they just 'feel right' – and because they have, we have learned to really trust our hearts ever more dutifully, every step of this joyous journey.

From the first pitch to the final edit of *Sattva*, we have really enjoyed 'the process' – it's been an atypically gentle, happy, flowing thing, most of it written very close to home, in a quiet, sun-filled café in the middle of Kentish woodland. Ah, we already cherish these memories. To our gorgeous, arms-wide-open Hay House family – Michelle Pilley, Jo Burgess, Sian Orrell: there really are no words significant enough to encompass our unending gratitude.

Amy Kiberd, who has since flown the HH nest, but who was truly instrumental in all of this – thank you. To Leanne, Debra, Diane,

Rachel, Clem, Elaine, Tom, Julie N. and Julie O. – for your vision, guidance, openness and hardest work in bringing this book to life and out into the world.

To beautiful soul, Alisha Rose Kruger, for creating essence-igniting magic with your sacred shapes – we are so happy to have connected with you. Your work is purest sattva.

To our parents, whose unconditional love is held in our hearts and splashed across these pages – we love you.

To our cheerleading and light-bearing friends for your supportive words and energy, and the team of wonder women at *Psychologies* magazine, led so graciously by Suzy (Sky) Walker – we love you all.

To our beautiful wellbeing community – at This Conscious Life, through Instagram and far beyond: we cherish our connections and are so thankful to you all for your encouragement.

To Dr David Frawley and Dr Vasant Lad, for their life's work and the sparks of wisdom that lit the first flames – and reminded us of not just who we really are at our essence, but also illuminated our path back there.

To all carriers and conduits of the shared and limitless love that knows no borders, walls or chosen people. And to you, dear reader – for inviting us into your life and reminding us, yet again, of the indistinguishability of you and me, us and them. Here, once more, we are all one.

Paul & Eminé

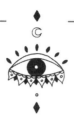

THE CLEARING

A year-long conscious living programme
to support your natural and seasonal
wellbeing, launching September 2019.

We'll meet you at The Clearing.

www.thisconsciouslife.co/theclearing

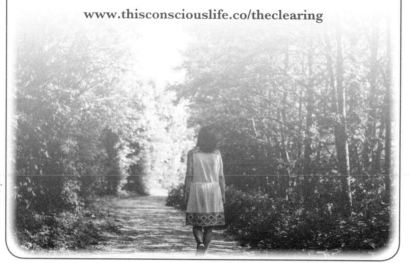

Aiste Saulyte

ABOUT THE AUTHORS

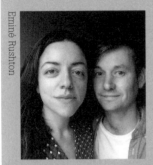

Eminé Kali Rushton and **Paul Rushton** are co-founders of This Conscious Life, an online journal that celebrates the joys of living consciously. Eminé is a Conscious Living columnist and writer, and was *Psychologies'* Wellbeing Director for nine years. Paul is a freelance food, travel and nature writer, and also a contributing editor at *Psychologies*. Eminé is also a qualified holistic therapist, and has studied Ayurvedic Healing with the American Institute of Vedic Studies, founded by Dr David Frawley.

Seven years ago Eminé and Paul left a busy London life behind for spring bluebells, autumn chestnuts and a ramshackle cottage in Kent. There they live with their two daughters, tending a small garden and local village allotment plot – a place to grow, heal and rest, naturally.

They try to keep life as simple as possible. It's not all cottage roses, but it is all underpinned by these pleasurable beliefs – that free and cheap can also be rich; simple is delightful; and natural can offer up the most powerful, plentiful and bountiful treasures of all.

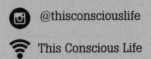

@thisconsciouslife

This Conscious Life

www.thisconsciouslife.co

Hay House Podcasts
Bring Fresh, Free Inspiration Each Week!

HAY HOUSE
Online Video Courses

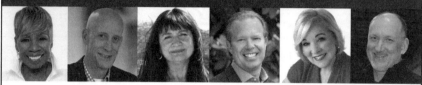

Your journey to a better life starts with figuring out which path is best for you. Hay House Online Courses provide guidance in mental and physical health, personal finance, telling your unique story, and so much more!

LEARN HOW TO:

- choose your words and actions wisely so you can tap into life's magic
- clear the energy in yourself and your environments for improved clarity, peace, and joy
- forgive, visualize, and trust in order to create a life of authenticity and abundance
- break free from the grip of narcissists and other energy vampires in your life
- sculpt your platform and your message so you get noticed by a publisher
- use the creative power of the quantum realm to create health and well-being

To find the guide for your journey,
visit www.HayHouseU.com.

HAY HOUSE
online learning

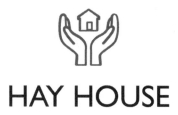

HAY HOUSE

Look within

Join the conversation about latest products,
events, exclusive offers and more.

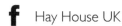 Hay House UK

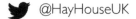 @HayHouseUK

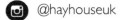 @hayhouseuk

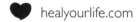 healyourlife.com

We'd love to hear from you!